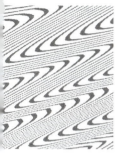

Electric and Magnetic Fields: Invisible Risks?

Electric and Magnetic Fields: Invisible Risks?

Leonard A. Sagan, MD

GORDON AND BREACH PUBLISHERS

Australia • Canada • China • France • Germany • India •
Japan • Luxembourg • Malaysia • The Netherlands • Russia •
Singapore • Switzerland • Thailand • United Kingdom

Emmaplain 5
1075 AW Amsterdam
The Netherlands

British Library Cataloguing in Publication Data

Sagan, Leonard A.
    Electric and magnetic fields : invisible risks?
    1.Electric fields – Physiological effect 2.Magnetic fields
    – Physiological effect 3.Electromagnetism – Physiological
    effect
    I.Title
    363.1'89

    ISBN   2–88449–217–8

CONTENTS

TABLES

FIGURES

FOREWORD

Americans display an extraordinary degree of ambivalence when it comes to taking personal risks. Surely no modern nation has as many extreme skiers, white-water rafters, urban skateboarders, or sport parachutists. Yet we resent having risks imposed on us by others, and display our affection for litigation at the "drop of a hat" when we suspect that someone else has put us in harm's way.

When it comes to the government's responsibility for our safety, we are caught up in confusion. No issue in our domestic politics is as capable of generating high expectations, high anxiety, and high dudgeon. On the one hand, we expect societal rules to protect us from every possible kind of covert hazard; on the other, we bridle at any effort on the part of government to interfere with what is immediately described as our "freedom of choice." It is, therefore, hardly surprising that regulation and regulatory reform have repeatedly been at the core of congressional policy debates. No single issue in the 1995 "Contract with America" produced hotter arguments than the Republican proposals to reduce the levels of environmental and health and safety regulations.

Public concern takes on an even sharper edge when the risk is a cancer risk. The politics of cancer is unusually powerful. It has attracted more federal research money than any other disease; it is the only illness to have had a "war" declared on it by a president of the United States and his administration. Just as cancer has political clout as an attraction for research funding, cancer causation—carcinogenesis—has dominated the political arena of health and safety regulation. It has led to special legislation: the Delaney Clause—a controversial provision over thirty years old that forbids residues in or on processed food of any amount of a pesticide known to cause cancer in man or laboratory animals . . . no matter how nominal the risk. Under the Delaney Clause also, the pesticide must "concentrate," i.e., become stronger during processing. Often criticized for its "zero tolerance" character, the Delaney Clause has proven politically durable largely because people have such profound dread of this disease.

Cancer has generated a long list of public "scares" that have led to new legislation or regulations. It is an all too familiar litany: Love Canal, DDT, Rocky Flats, diethylstilbestrol, polychlorinated biphenyls. Along with it, however, goes another list, much less familiar—the list of scares that somehow vanished. The pesticide Alar, backyard barbecued hamburgers, radio-frequency cellular telephones, and your morning coffee have all been declared as hazards with significant media fanfare, only to drop off the horizon of public concern.

As a result, there is an authentic public confusion as to what is worth worrying about. A spate of recent literature reassures us that most of our worries are due to scare-merchants or publicity-seeking scientists determined, for their own reasons, to persuade us that we are at risk. Yet new and troubling revelations continue to crop up, and they are sometimes real causes for concern—often enough, at any rate, to keep us alert though skeptical.

One of the best publicized of the "new worries" is the cancer-causing potential of electrical and magnetic fields (EMF). It is almost a textbook case in the application of public policy in a domain of scientific uncertainty and popular furor. Partly because of some tantalizing scientific findings, and with a substantial assist from the efforts of a journalist named Paul Brodeur, the possibility that EMF might cause human cancers of several types has become a public health issue of international concern. Scientific groups and public bodies in half a dozen countries have studied the problem and issued reports. Legislatures and assemblies in the United States have debated the issue and proposed regulatory solutions. Schools have been relocated at substantial public expense in order to distance students from transmission lines and other EMF sources. And new findings—and pseudo-findings—on this subject continue to command intense public attention.

It is easy to understand why people are confused. On the one hand, there are persuasive accounts of cancer "clusters"—local concentrations of cases that are of great concern to those in the neighborhood. These incidents, publicized effectively by Brodeur and other journalists, raise intense anxiety. It seems impossible to believe that for any health end-point, it is a statistical certainty that some neighborhood will show an occasional, dramatic excess. Set against these incidents are unconvincing reassurances from public officials, or pronouncements from expert groups—like the American Physical Society—to the effect that there is no scientific basis for such a phenomenon. The former are often treated with the skepticism reserved for efforts at political comfort. The latter are seriously attended, but most thoughtful people are skeptical of claims that say, in effect, "we know of no theoretically possible cause so the observations must be wrong."

Physician and radiation biologist Leonard Sagan has turned a thoughtful eye to this difficult muddle in science and public policy. The evaluation of risk in this situation depends on a careful, dispassionate analysis of the data. The question of what risk EMF poses for the public has to be answered, in the end, by good science. The requisite research, however, occupies two quite different arenas. One is that of basic science: what cellular mechanisms or effects on the central nervous system might account for a health effect of electrical and magnetic fields? The second is the population-based discipline of epidemiology: is there significant evidence, after all other factors have been eliminated from the situation, of a correlation between EMF exposure and the incidence of a particular type of cancer?

Dr. Sagan makes it clear that for now—in the absence of clearer evidence at the level of biological mechanism—the case must rest on convincing demonstrations of an association between exposure and outcome in populations of real people. Much of this book is thus devoted to a summary and analysis of the large number of epidemiological and occupational health evaluations that have been done in several countries.

This approach is an indispensable one for the intelligent citizen who is concerned for the public health, but also committed to the development of sound policies. The EMF controversy is clouded with ambiguity, and it is an arena in which wise decision making is unusually difficult. Therein lies its interest—because in those respects it resembles many of the most challenging problems we face. If readers are left in doubt about the outcome, they are in good company. At least, in facing up to the same uncertainties our public officials face, they will understand the difficulties under which these officials regularly labor. And perhaps they will not be so tempted to

PREFACE

This book is about a source of possible environmental risk—exposure to the electric and magnetic fields (EMF) around power lines and electrical appliances. Studies show that over 50 percent of the American public are aware of this research. About half this number are aware of a link between EMF and cancer, and more than half of these (approximately 10 percent of the total) feel that the risk is somewhat serious or very serious (EEI94). However, the majority of respondents who are aware of the issue feel that the risk is uncertain, and that more research is necessary before regulations are instituted.

Still, many people are deeply concerned about these fields. Mothers worry about their children's exposure, and because of this concern, school boards are often besieged with questions about the safety of their schools. The real estate industry must contend with these worries, and electrical utilities often have difficulty in siting new power lines or substations. The reassuring words of scientific bodies, asserting that the risks are unproven, do little to quiet public anxieties.

One important reason for public apprehension is the considerable controversy concerning EMF risks among members of the scientific community. For every expert who asserts that there is no reason for worry, there is another expert who expresses deep anxieties about these risks. How can this be? How can good scientists examining the same studies come to different conclusions? The answer is that different scientists utilize different rules for reaching decisions. Some public health officials are likely to be overly cautious in interpreting possible EMF risks, arguing that it is better to err on the side of prudence. Other scientists, who might be called scientific purists, are likely to demand rigorous evidence of risk before accepting the existence of those risks.

For example, although many epidemiological studies show some evidence of a small risk from exposure to EMF, other studies, as we shall see, do not . This can be interpreted in two ways: a small risk exists, but cannot always be demonstrated; or the studies suggesting risks are flawed. Opinions among scientists vary about what to do under these circumstances.

At the same time, because of the arcane nature of risk assessment, much of the general public has difficulty reaching independent judgments about the possible risks of EMF. Most people know little about these fields or how to interpret the many health studies of exposed populations that frequently appear in our newspapers or on our televisions. Original studies are not easily available to members of the public.

What Is EMF?

What are these fields and how does one evaluate the validity of the claims that there are risks to health from exposure? The remainder of this book will explore these issues in some detail, but this preface presents a bird's-eye view.

The fields are invisible; if you drive an automobile under high-voltage transmission lines with the car radio playing, you may be aware of an electrical field because of the noisy interference heard on the radio. If you walk under such lines, you may feel a slight tingling of the skin. These same fields, at much lower intensities, surround all electrical equipment, including hair dryers, television sets, electric stoves, and all other common household appliances. Fields will be discussed in more detail in chapter 2.

"Electromagnetic" or "Electric *and* Magnetic"?

Electromagnetic fields carry energy through space. These fields can be represented as waves with a broad range of frequencies (Figure Pr.I).

As the frequency of the waves increases, the energy of those waves increases. For example, at the highest frequencies—X rays and gamma rays—the energies of these waves are sufficient to break chemical bonds, separating electrons from their atoms, thus producing electrically charged ions. For this reason, X rays and gamma rays are said to be "ionizing." Frequencies lower than those that are ionizing are sometimes referred to as "non-ionizing." As the frequency decreases, the waves assume different properties. Visible light, heat, microwaves, and radio waves represent increasingly lower ener-

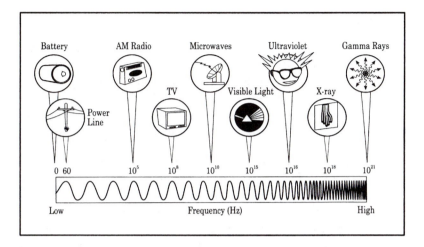

Figure Pr.I   Electromagnetic Spectrum

gies. Finally, at the lowest end of the spectrum, we come to the frequency of electric power—60 cycles per second, referred to as
power-frequency—where the energy is insufficient to break chemical bonds or even to heat tissue. At power-frequency, the wave crests
are thousands of miles apart, whereas the space separating crests of
X rays is smaller than the nucleus of an atom. Electromagnetic waves
at the higher frequencies are always associated with both electric
and magnetic fields—they are inseparable. At very low frequencies
such as power-frequencies, however, the electric field and magnetic
field can, under certain conditions, exist independently; i.e., a 60-Hz
electric field and a 60-Hz magnetic field can each exist without the
other. Therefore, for these low frequencies, appropriate terminology
is electric *and* magnetic fields, rather than electromagnetic fields. Accordingly, some people prefer the abbreviation E/MF, using the
slash for *and*. This distinction is not just a matter of scientific snob-
bery; as we shall see, there are many situations, particularly in the
laboratory, where either electric field or magnetic field conditions
are examined independently. The use of the term *electric and magnetic
fields* (EMF) keeps us cognizant of the distinction. Although there
may be valid reasons for objecting to the use of EMF as jargon for
power frequency electric and magnetic fields, the term has become widely used and attempts to avoid it would be awkward and pedantic.

Evaluating Risks

All of us are exposed to numerous risks from a great variety of sources ranging from natural disasters—lightning, fires, earthquakes, floods—to illnesses—including fatal illnesses—and accidents—drowning, gunshot wounds, automobile and airplane accidents. Whether consciously or unconsciously, we make judgments about these risks, their magnitude, and what to do about them.

Some examples: you notice that the treads on the tires of your car are wearing a little thin. You know that such tires increase the hazard of driving. You consider the cost of replacing the tires; you also consider how much expendable cash you have on hand. You might also factor into the decision other safety needs—relining the brakes may be a more important need than the tires. Also, safety needs may compete with other family needs. The children need new clothes for school—maybe that takes precedence over tires or brakes. In making such decisions, you are engaging in risk assessment and risk management.

Risk assessment may arise in a medical environment. Your child has a low-grade fever and is complaining of a painful ear; should you take the child to a doctor? There will certainly be a wait—possibly some expense; and what do you do with your other children who are sleeping? At this point, you have to make a decision about risk. The child has had, or has not had, other episodes like this; it is snowing outside and there is some risk in driving. Here is a real problem in risk assessment. Generally, the data available for each of these contingencies is limited; nevertheless, a decision must be made.

Risks from exposures to various chemical and physical agents in the air, water, and food supply are difficult problems—problems in decision making with which most of us are ill-equipped to deal. I refer to substances of industrial origin, such as pesticides or naturally occurring agents, such as dietary cholesterol, that in small quantities or low concentrations are alleged to result in subtle increases in common diseases such as cancer and heart disease. Indeed, even environmental scientists often have difficulty in characterizing these risks, particularly when the risks are small and uncertain; the scientific methods available to us for estimating such risks are far from precise. Are the reported risks real or merely artifacts in the data? What, then, are lay members of the public to do, when, for example, there are reports of cancer among children who eat hot dogs? (Sa94, Pe94b) What is one to make of these reports?

If the reported risks are real, i.e., confirmed, are they big or small? How do the risks of living near a nuclear power plant compare with the risks of cigarette smoking, eating peanut butter—said to contain cancer-producing substances—or using an electric blanket?

There are systematic means of estimating risks. The discipline that attempts to identify and quantify risks is called risk assessment. The techniques of risk assessment are not widely taught or understood, even within the scientific community. One of the important goals of this book is to provide an introduction to these techniques.

Risks from Exposures to EMF: Real or Unreal?

The issue of possible risks from EMF is important, as all of us are exposed at some level. Even if the risk is small, as is the case with childhood cancer, it may, nonetheless, be so serious and so tragic a risk that it warrants great concern.

Risk assessment is not easy; it involves some understanding of epidemiology—the science of studying disease among human populations. It also requires some insight into laboratory sciences. What can we learn from studying the responses of cells and animals, and what do these studies tell us about cancer? This book assumes that the reader has little knowledge of these disciplines; therefore, there are introductory chapters on these and other disciplines involved in evaluating risks from EMF.

In many chapters, special text sections present background material that may not be useful to some readers. Such material is contained in side bars and can easily be skipped. Although the book is not meant to provide a comprehensive review of all relevant EMF literature, it is intended to provide sufficient information for the reader to make some judgment about the possible risks of EMF, as well as to acquire those skills necessary to assess other environmental risks.

Who Should Read This Book?

The medical community—both clinicians and public health officials who need information regarding environmental risks to guide their own decision making as well as to counsel patients.

Members of the electrical utility industry—all of those who are responsible for the planning, design, and construction of electrical conductors should be familiar with the evidence of possible risk from EMF. So, too, should those in public information, who must be prepared to answer questions regarding this area of research.

Electrical workers—who are themselves frequently exposed to electric and magnetic fields and who are also called upon by friends, clients, and neighbors to answer questions about possible health effects.

The regulatory/legislative community—who must make policy decisions regarding possible consequences of threats to the public health.

Science writers and teachers—who are responsible for reporting this body of data.

Members of the real estate industry—who must be able to answer questions from prospective buyers regarding possible health effects of environmental exposures, particularly from nearby power lines or substations.

Lawyers—who must evaluate claims regarding possible harmful health effects from EMF exposures.

School board members and educators—who are responsible for providing safe environments for the children in their charge.

Organization of This Book

The book is organized into seven parts.

Part One (chapter 1) contains introductory material. Chapter 1 reviews the more recent history of the emergence, over the past thirty years, of the EMF issue as a possible threat to health.

Part Two (chapters 2–3) provides background material on the electrical power system and the occurrence and measurement of the electrical and magnetic fields found near conductors of electricity. Chapter 2 describes the design of the electrical system and the characteristics of the electric and magnetic fields they produce. Chapter 3 describes the means of assessing human exposures to these fields, as necessary to the conduct of epidemiological studies.

Part Three (chapters 4–5) addresses the issue of how EMF might interact with tissues and cells to produce health effects. Chapter 4 discusses some of the proposed mechanisms that might explain the influence of EMF on tissues, while chapter 5 reviews the laboratory studies intended to examine some of the proposed mechanisms

Part Four (chapters 6–8) introduces the reader to the methods of risk assessment and, in particular, the science of epidemiology—the major source of the evidence linking electrical conductors to human disease, particularly cancer. Chapter 6 provides a brief review of the practice and methodology of risk assessment. Chapter 7 is an historical introduction to the discussion of epidemiological methods in chapter 8.

Part Five (chapters 9–11) describes the two collections of epidemiological studies linking EMF to cancer —studies of cancer and exposures in the home in chapter 9 and studies of cancer among electrical workers in chapter 10. Chapter 11 addresses the issue of cancer clusters.

Part Six (chapters 12–13) describes the studies of EMF and diseases other than cancer—reproductive studies in chapter 12 and neurobehavioral studies in chapter 13.

Part Seven (chapters 14–16) attempts to bring the information in the previous chapters to bear on some key questions:

- How large a risk could EMF exposure pose, if the risk is real? (chapter 14)

- What are the views of scientific review committees on the risks of EMF? (chapter 15)

- What options exist for the management of EMF exposures? (chapter 16)

References included in the text utilize the name of the first author, of which the first two letters of the last name precede the date of publication. For example, a publication of Benjamin Franklin, 1780, would be shown as (Fr80).

A Glossary is at the end of the book. When words found in the glossary appear in the text for the first time, the word is shown in **bold type**.

ACKNOWLEDGMENTS

The purpose of this book is to provide information needed by non-experts to make a judgment about possible health effects of the electric and magnetic fields that surround electrical conductors. To explain the many issues involved in such an evaluation properly, the book could have been written in one of two ways: either many experts could have been invited to write individual chapters, or a single author might alone attempt the task. Each method has advantages and disadvantages. The advantage of the multiple-author technique is that each of the authors has the expertise to write his or her own chapter unassisted and in an authoritative manner. The disadvantage is that such a multi-authored book is inevitably uneven and often repetitive. The single-author strategy overcomes this disadvantage; however, no single individual can have mastered all of the many facets of this complex subject.

The remedy available to the single author is to call on individual experts to review chapters, assist in maintaining technical accuracy, point out the biases that inevitably creep into the text, and identify significant research that has not been taken into consideration. I have been very fortunate with the extraordinary generosity of the many experts, whose names appear below, who have read and commented extensively on each chapter of the book. I hasten to add that the reviews were generally carried out in early stages of writing—the present manuscript may appear quite unfamiliar to reviewers who saw earlier drafts. The reviewers certainly bear no responsibility for the final manuscript. All of the errors are solely my responsibility.

Reviewers to whom I should like to express my great appreciation are: Eleanor and Robert Adair, A. A. Afifi, Larry Anderson, William Bailey, Robert Banks, Robert Brent, Philip Cole, John Dunlap, Donald Justesen, William Kaune, Robert Kavet, Ralph Keeney, Leeka Kheifets, Richard Lovely, Kenneth McLeod, M. Granger Morgan, Raymond Neutra, Robert Olson, John Peters, Charles Polk, Charles

Rafferty, Kenneth Rothman, Richard Stephens, Nancy Wertheimer, Chris Whipple, Detlov Von Winterfeld, and Frank Young.

Three reviewers—Stanley Sussman, George Hidy, and Kenneth Foster—read the entire manuscript and deserve special thanks. Susan Kimber, among other more important things, changed all the "whiches" to "thats" and "thats" to "whiches"—for which I am very grateful.

Much of this book was written while I was employed as Senior Medical Scientist at the Electric Power Research Institute (EPRI) in Palo Alto, California. The staff of the EMF Health Effects Program has been of enormous help to me in understanding the many difficult and technical issues associated with the study of the possible health effects of exposure to electric and magnetic fields. I am grateful for their support. I am also grateful to the EPRI for allowing me the freedom to write this book. Neither the EPRI, nor any member of the EPRI, nor any person acting on its behalf, however, offers any warranties, express or implied, for the contents of this book, or assumes any liability associated with or resulting from the selection or use of or reliance on this book or any information disclosed in this book. The opinions and positions expressed here are strictly my own, and should not be taken as the opinions or positions of the EPRI.

I
INTRODUCTION

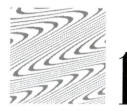

1

Recent Emergence of the EMF Issue

In this chapter, the EMF health issue will be traced as it developed over the past thirty or so years from that time when the possibility that EMF could cause health effects was considered totally implausible to the present, when there are some who are now convinced that health effects of EMF exposure do occur, and many at least willing to entertain such a possibility.

Soviet Studies of Electrical Workers

Perhaps the first hint of possible harm from exposure to EMF arose from studies conducted in the Soviet Union in the 1960s (Ko72). These focused on utility workers, particularly those employed at stations where higher **voltages** are transformed to lower voltages (**substations**). Studies of the health of these employees found a higher than expected rate of symptoms such as sleeplessness, headache, and upper respiratory symptoms. Although subsequent studies in several Western countries (including Germany, France, Canada, and

3

the United States) failed to confirm these findings (Br85) , the Soviet studies were important because they were the first to raise questions about health effects from EMF exposure.

These early epidemiological studies, and the laboratory studies that were conducted in parallel, were designed to assess possible biological and health effects of <u>electric</u> fields. One reason for concern regarding electric fields was that electric utilities were considering **transmission lines** of increasingly higher voltages and the electric field (the magnitude of which is related to voltage) would be higher for these new designs; could these exposures pose risks to human health?

Project Seafarer

When, in the early 1970s, the U.S. Navy proposed the construction of a worldwide communications system known as Seafarer, fears arose about the possibility of health effects among residents of the state of Wisconsin where the facility was to be built. The system was to operate at frequencies near the power frequency. Although the Navy insisted that the system would be harmless to human populations, many members of the public were nevertheless concerned—there were relatively few studies of possible human health effects from prolonged exposures to such fields.

The Seafarer controversy resulted in the commissioning of a number of studies by such prestigious agencies as the National Academy of Sciences, and in extensive biological investigations. The danger of these fields was never proven. Eventually, a smaller system known as "Project ELF" was constructed.

An Ambassador Becomes Ill in Moscow

Another episode from the 1970s, this time involving fields at frequencies much higher than 60 Hz, was the detection of intensive Soviet electronic surveillance of the U.S. Embassy in Moscow, resulting in concerns that this was producing health effects among embassy personnel. While the Soviet use of microwave surveillance had been known to U.S. intelligence agencies for many years, there was little concern until the development of **leukemia** in the American Ambassador, Walter Stoessel, and reports of suspicious alterations in the blood counts of some Americans who had previously served in the

Moscow embassy. The concern spurred an epidemiological survey conducted by the late Abraham Lillienfeld of Johns Hopkins University. His extensive study, completed in 1978, produced no evidence of health effects from exposures experienced in the embassy (Po92). Although this episode did not involve power frequency exposures, nor did it produce evidence of harm from exposure, publicity regarding the incident nevertheless again served to raise public suspicion of possible health effects following exposure to non-ionizing radiation.

The Wertheimer-Leeper Study

The study that first brought the issue of EMF to the widespread attention of the public and the scientific community was the childhood cancer study conducted by Nancy Wertheimer and Ed Leeper. The study was conducted in the 1970s and published in the American Journal of Epidemiology in 1979 (We 79). Because of the importance of this study, it will be discussed in detail in Chapter 9. Suffice it to state here, the Wertheimer-Leeper study did several things: most importantly, it raised the possibility that EMF might increase deaths from cancer, particularly among children. No previous scientific findings had hinted at that possibility. Second, the study was designed to assess the <u>magnetic field</u> component of EMF, thus shifting attention from the electric field component that had previously dominated scientific attention. That emphasis on magnetic fields remains with us today. Third, the study drew attention to power lines as a possibly important source of power-frequency magnetic fields.

To study magnetic fields, Wertheimer-Leeper devised a system known as "wire coding" that permitted researchers to achieve an estimation of indoor magnetic field levels without actually entering the home. Since the magnetic field around a power line depends upon the amount of power being carried on the line and decreases in a known manner with distance, the two investigators devised a system that allowed them to estimate the indoor magnetic field level by (1) measuring the distance between the home and the power lines, and (2) making judgments of the power being carried by counting the size and number of conductors on those poles. This methodology is based on the assumption that neighboring power lines are the major source of exposure within residential structures. In Chapter 3, the validity of these assumptions will be discussed.

While the Wertheimer-Leeper study attracted a good deal of attention, it also met with a good deal of skepticism. There were a number of reasons for this skepticism, the first of which was the uncertainty regarding the means of assessing the magnetic field exposure: is the wire code an adequate surrogate for magnetic fields? Secondly, there was no known mechanism which could begin to explain how these very weak fields might produce significant health effects, and thirdly, a similar study published shortly after failed to confirm the results of the Wertheimer-Leeper study (Fu80). Much of this skepticism remains today.

Another noteworthy feature of the Wertheimer-Leeper report stems from what appeared almost as an aside in the report—a single table and a brief statement that **electrical workers** also appeared to have a small excess of cancer. This study spawned a relatively large and continuing series of similar studies of cancer among electrical workers. This series of occupational investigations will be reviewed in some detail in Chapter 10.

New York Power Line Project

In 1975, the New York Power Authority proposed the construction of a 765-thousand volt (765 kV) transmission line designed for the purpose of bringing electric power from Canada into New York State. Because of strong public opposition, extensive hearings were held on all environmental consequences of the line, and among the issues raised were possible health effects from exposure to electric and magnetic fields. The hearings lasted for a total of three years, and produced a record of 36,000 pages of testimony. A settlement was reached that permitted construction of the line. An agreement was also reached that the New York electric utilities fund a five-year research project, to be conducted under the direction of the New York State Department of Health.

The New York-sponsored research program conducted 16 individual EMF studies, the majority of them finding no convincing evidence of possible health effects. One, however, the only epidemiological study, turned out to be a second important landmark in the development of interest in magnetic fields and human cancer. This project, conducted in Denver by David Savitz and colleagues, was a study of childhood cancer clearly meant to further investigate the validity of the earlier Wertheimer-Leeper study. The

Savitz study results appeared consistent with the earlier Wertheimer-Leeper study results (Sa88).

Another feature of the Savitz study was that it was the first to measure magnetic fields within the home. Those measurements gave different results than those obtained with the use of the wiring code. The relationship of these two indices of magnetic field exposures with cancer will be discussed in Chapter 9.

Subsequent Studies

Following the Savitz report, two subsequent studies of childhood cancer and EMF attracted a good deal of attention from the public as well as from the scientific community. These were conducted in Los Angeles, California, (Lo91) and in Stockholm, Sweden (Fe93). Both have been interpreted as consistent with the Wertheimer-Leeper and Savitz studies in suggesting increased **risks** among children living near power lines; however, neither of these subsequent studies, in which magnetic fields were carefully measured, showed a significant association between cancer risk and measured magnetic fields. As shall be seen later, in the absence of increased magnetic field levels, the explanation for increased cancer risk among some (but not all) populations living near power lines remains an enigma even today.

Public Awareness

Over the past few years, press coverage of the EMF effects issue has greatly increased. Most prominent among the writers following the issue is Paul Brodeur, an investigative journalist who has published in *The New Yorker* since 1958. His earlier writings, first serialized in *The New Yorker*, and then published in book form, focused on the health effects of asbestos, but he wrote extensively on non-ionizing radiation as well. On this latter subject, his early concern with microwave radiation resulted in the book, *The Zapping of America*. More recently, he has turned his attention to power-frequency exposures and health, and these writings have undoubtedly been a major factor in bringing possible EMF risk to the attention of the public.

While not a scientist, Brodeur interprets the scientific literature as showing definite health effects from EMF exposure and claims that these hazards are well known to utilities, government agencies and other officials, but have been systematically suppressed. His views are extensively described in his two books, *Currents of Death: Power Lines, Computer Terminals, and the Attempt to Cover Up Their Threat to Your Health* (Br89), and *The Great Power-Line Cover-Up: How the Utilities and the Government Are Trying to Hide the Cancer Hazards Posed by Electromagnetic Fields* (Br93c).

Because of growing public concern, three different committees of the U.S. Congress have held hearings on possible health effects of EMF. While none has led to regulatory legislation, the Energy Bill of 1992 authorized a $65-million research program, to be funded by both public and private sectors, and to be expended over a five-year period.

Summary

Over the past thirty years or so, a variety of reports related to possible health effects of low frequency electric and magnetic fields have appeared that have heightened both public and scientific interest in this area of research. The remainder of this book will attempt to explore the scientific basis for this interest; what do we know, and why are there uncertainties?

II

ELECTRIC POWER, EMF, AND EXPOSURE

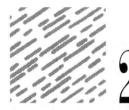

2

Electric Power and EMF

An examination of possible health effects of electric and magnetic fields requires an understanding of electricity, of the fields that surround electrical conductors, and of the sources of those fields in the residential environment and in the workplace.

This chapter will begin with a description of basic electrical concepts (e.g., voltage and current), summarize the operation of electrical power systems, and describe the fields that surround electrical conductors. Methodology for measurement of fields will be described in chapter 3. More extensive and more technical treatment of these subjects can be found in three recent books (FR94, Hi95, Ho95).

About Volts, Watts, Amps, and Hertz

Modern electrical utility systems employ various means to generate electrical power. Utilizing steam or water power, a turbine spins an electrical generator, moving electrical conductors through a magnetic field, inducing an electric current in the conductors.

In high school physics classes, *voltage* is frequently compared with the *pressure* in your water system; the comparison is a very useful one.

11

Both the voltage and the water pressure exist regardless of whether electricity or water flows. Similarly, *current* has its parallel with the *rate* of water flow. No matter how many homes are drawing electric current, voltage will remain nearly constant, while the current will increase or decrease as utility customers turn on appliances and motors.

Voltage is expressed in units of volts (V). Our homes are wired for 115 and 230 V, while the electric power lines that transport electricity operate at thousands of volts (or kilovolts, kV). Electric current is expressed in units of amperes (A), sometimes called amps for short. The amount of electric *power*, expressed in units of watts (W), is related to the voltage multiplied by the current. The same amount of power can be transported either at high voltage and low current, or at low voltage and high current. At an electrical substation, the voltage is reduced (or "stepped down") while the current rises—the amount of power is essentially unchanged. Those relationships can be expressed as follows:

$$Power = voltage \ X \ current$$

It is possible to generate and transmit electrical energy as a direct, or non- alternating, current (generally referred to as dc). DC currents do not alternate in direction, but always move in the same direction. Batteries provide dc current; your flashlight and your automobile's electrical system operate on dc current. U.S. utility systems, however, generate electrical energy as alternating current (**ac**) at a frequency of 60 cycles per second (also known as **hertz**, or Hz). At some places in the world, such as in parts of Japan and in Europe, power is generated at 50 Hz

---

Edison, Tesla, and Westinghouse

When commercial electrical distribution first began in the last quarter of the nineteenth century, Thomas Edison strongly endorsed the use of direct current for domestic and industrial use. However, a dispute arose with Nikola Tesla (1856–1943), a proponent of alternating current. Tesla, born in Croatia, was an inventor, an eccentric, and an engineering genius. Like Edison, his fertile imagination was the source of many of the every-day technologies upon which we depend today—including the radio. Tesla's name was given to the SI unit of magnetic flux density widely used in Europe (Ch81).

At the beginning of the electrical era, there were obvious advantages to ac generation. For example, **transformers** do not work with direct current; therefore, changing voltages becomes complicated. Moreover, there was at that time no practical motor that could operate on alternating current. Tesla developed such a motor. In collaboration with George Westinghouse, ac systems went head to head with Edison's dc system. Edison began a vicious propaganda campaign, claiming that ac systems were dangerous. To emphasize his point, Edison staged electrocutions of stray animals ("Westinghoused"), and is said to have been instrumental in arranging a criminal execution by electrocution at the state penitentiary (Pe94a).

Because of the greater efficiency and lower costs of ac power, dc power was rapidly superseded by ac and is now used almost exclusively throughout the world, with the exception of a few high-voltage, long-distance transmission lines.

The Utility Power Network

Whereas the voltage in your home is 115 V, electrical utilities transmit electrical power over long distances at much higher voltages, often at hundreds of thousands of volts (Figure 2.I) The simple reason is that it is more efficient, since energy lost (as heat) in transmission is proportional to the square of the current. Since, as indicated by the power formula (shown earlier), current is related to power divided by voltage, higher-voltage systems lose less energy for a fixed amount of energy transfer.

If the power were carried at low voltages and high currents, very large conductors would be required to provide the same efficiency. For example, the power carried from a 1000-MW power station would require many conductors on multiple lines rather than just one line.

At high voltages, it is necessary for safety and engineering purposes to carry conductors high up on transmission towers. In the United States, high-voltage transmission may vary from 50 through 765 kV. Since power is often generated at remote sites, the transmission towers can be often be seen crossing mountains and fields, carrying energy to cities and towns, or, in utility parlance, "load centers." There are about 350,000 miles of such transmission lines; in the United States. Generally, no homes or other occupied structures

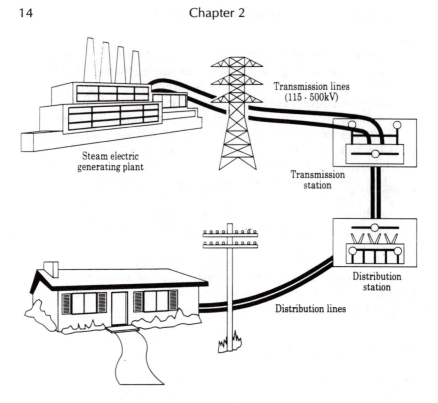

Transmission lines
(115 - 500kV)

Steam electric
generating plant

Transmission
station

Distribution
station

Distribution lines

Figure 2.1   Utility Power Network (Source: EPRI)

are permitted in the rights of way below these lines, and the width of the **right-of-way** is controlled by engineering design and by safety codes. In many countries, there are no prohibitions on the use of land beneath transmission lines.

The route of a transmission line will terminate at a **substation**, where the energy is parceled into smaller blocks, at lower voltages, to be carried on *distribution lines* to commercial and industrial customers, as well as to residential neighborhoods. At the substation the transmission voltage is reduced with a transformer to a lower voltage suitable for distribution via primary distribution lines that generally carry 4 to 35 kV. The distribution lines are strung on poles (generally wooden) that usually also support telephone lines, and are common sights in most communities; in newer subdivisions, distribution lines may be underground. It is estimated that there are about two million miles of distribution lines in the United States.

The voltage of primary distribution lines would not be safe to use in the home or workplace; therefore, voltage is again reduced by distribution transformers to 115/230 volts for residential use. These transformers, generally cylindrical in shape, are seen mounted near the top of utility poles. There are millions of these in service throughout the United States.

A **transformer** consists of a core of magnetic material (e.g., iron) around which are wrapped two coils of wire, one called the primary and the other called the secondary. The lines providing the electrical energy to the transformer feed the primary, and that energy is transferred through the magnetic core to the secondary.

The relationship of the voltage developed at the secondary to the voltage fed into the primary depends on the number of times the coils from each are wrapped on the magnetic core. If the numbers are equal, then the voltage at the secondary will equal the voltage at the primary. If the secondary coil is wrapped half as many times as the primary, the secondary will develop half the voltage applied to the primary. In this case, the transformer has *stepped down* the voltage.

Once current has flowed through an electrical device, it no longer is capable of doing work; it has expended its energy. Again, an analogy to water is helpful. Water raised above sea level in a dam is capable of spinning a turbine; water that has flowed to sea level has exhausted its energy and cannot be used to spin a turbine. The electrical analogy to sea level is called "ground potential." After current has been used, it flows out of a home and returns to the utility system.

Electric distribution lines to your home include two wire conductors carrying electricity into the house, and a conductor, called the neutral, which normally carries return current back to the utility system. However, national electrical codes require that this neutral conductor be grounded to your plumbing system as well; therefore, these weak neutral or "ground currents" may also find their way back to the utility system through the metallic water pipe that connects a home to the water main in the street. This connection serves as a very good conductor to the earth and is very important to the reduction of the risk of electrical shock or fire from short circuits.

"Fields"

We can experience the physiological effects of electricity either through direct contact with conductors, as when we touch an electrical appliance that is not well grounded (producing a "shock"), or by passing through a space in which there is an electrical or magnetic "field." What is a field?

In general, a field is a physical quantity that takes on different values at different points in space. One kind of field with which we have continuous and intimate contact is the earth's gravitational field. The field exerts a gravitational force on each of us that attracts us to the earth's surface and thereby keeps us from floating freely into space. The force weakens with distance from the earth to a point at which space travelers become essentially weightless.

Turning to the subject of this book, electric and magnetic fields are found everywhere in the vicinity where electricity is being conducted. They are not unique to high-voltage overhead transmission lines but exist in every residence, school, or workplace that receives electrical service. Fields in such locations arise from the electric distribution lines outside homes and buildings, as well as from indoor wiring and from appliances. These appliances may include electric stoves, electric washers and dryers, computer terminals, televisions, and electric blankets.

Electric and magnetic fields associated with the use of electricity share certain analogous properties with gravitational fields; they occupy space, decrease in intensity with increasing distance from their sources, and exert actions (or forces) at a distance (electric and magnetic rather than gravitational).

While electric and magnetic fields generally occur together, they can vary independently. The following two paragraphs describe the characteristics of the two kinds of fields.

Electric Fields From Electric Power Systems

Since the magnitude of electric fields is related to voltage (the units are volts per meter—V/m) the highest electric fields will be found around high-voltage transmission lines. Typical electric field levels in a home are a few volts per meter, whereas near a transmission line, the levels may be in the range of a few thousand volts per meter (kV/m).

Some of the characteristics of electric fields are as follows:

Electric fields *can be measured* with a simple meter.

They are *easily shielded* by walls, trees, or homes; therefore, electric fields indoors may be quite different (lower) than the fields outdoors under transmission lines.

Since the electric utility carefully regulates the voltage at which they generate power, electric fields around power lines and household appliances will be quite *constant* throughout the day or year, whether power is being conducted or not. Even when all appliances in your home are turned off and there is no flow of electricity, the electric fields in your home will be unaffected —just as when you turn off the water to your faucet, the pressure within the water pipe is unaffected.

Magnetic Fields in Homes

Magnetic fields are quite a different thing from electric fields. Unlike the constant electric fields, magnetic fields vary with the amount of current being drawn. For example, when you come home from work or school and turn on the electric range or other electric appliances, the *current* flowing in your home increases, as do the magnetic fields. That is because the magnitude of these fields is determined by current flow. As shown in Figure 2.II, only when an appliance is switched on will the ac magnetic field appear.

Typically, the magnetic fields around utility lines will rise in the late afternoon, fall to low levels in the middle of the night, and then begin to rise in the early morning as utility customers awaken and turn on appliances.

Unlike electric fields, magnetic fields cannot easily be shielded, and therefore will penetrate structures. Magnetic fields from outside sources, such as outdoor power lines or equipment, may sometimes be the dominant source of fields indoors, although it is not always easy to distinguish between indoor and outdoor sources of fields, i.e. to determine whether the fields measured within a home originate within or from outside sources.

Magnetic fields are most commonly expressed in units known as **Gauss** (after the German mathematician Karl Friedrich Gauss, 1777–1855). In the usual domestic or work environment, magnetic field levels are commonly a small fraction of one Gauss; the milligauss (mG), a thousandth of a Gauss, is therefore more convenient for measurements of residential magnetic fields. Another unit for magnetic fields, the Tesla, is far more often used in Europe. One Tesla

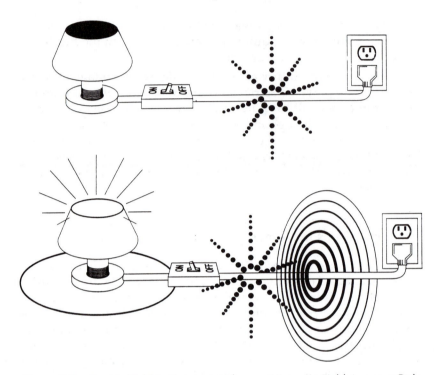

Figure 2.II   Electric Field is Constant, Whereas Magnetic Field Appears Only When Current is Flowing (Source: EPRI)

is equivalent to 10,000 Gauss, one millitesla is equivalent to 10 Gauss, and one microtesla is equivalent to 10 milligauss.

Magnetic fields measured more than a few feet from appliances in most homes are on the order of 1 mG or less. Differences among and within homes will depend on how the home is wired, the use of appliances, the proximity of the home to power lines, the amount of power carried on these lines, and the configuration of the conductors. Near high-voltage power lines, magnetic field levels may rarely be as high as 100 mG or more. Other locations where high magnetic fields may be found are near household appliances and in the workplace where electric power is used. Near welding equipment, for example, intermittent magnetic fields several hundred or even thousands of milligauss can be measured. A comparison of magnetic field strengths at varying distances around common household appliances is shown in Figure 2.III.

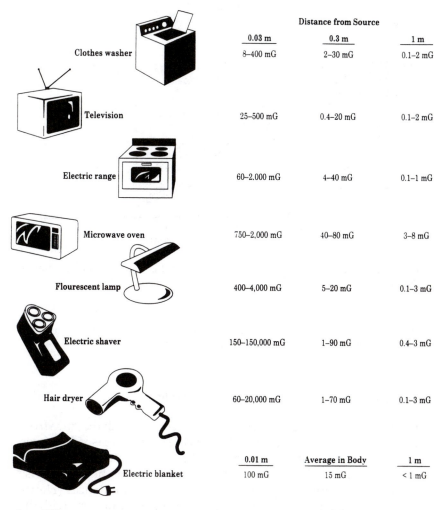

	Distance from Source		
	0.03 m	0.3 m	1 m
Clothes washer	8–400 mG	2–30 mG	0.1–2 mG
Television	25–500 mG	0.4–20 mG	0.1–2 mG
Electric range	60–2.000 mG	4–40 mG	0.1–1 mG
Microwave oven	750–2,000 mG	40–80 mG	3–8 mG
Flourescent lamp	400–4,000 mG	5–20 mG	0.1–3 mG
Electric shaver	150–150,000 mG	1–90 mG	0.4–3 mG
Hair dryer	60–20,000 mG	1–70 mG	0.1–3 mG

	0.01 m	Average in Body	1 m
Electric blanket	100 mG	15 mG	< 1 mG

Source: EPRI

Figure 2.III Magnetic Field Levels Near Household Appliances (Source: EPRI)

In a nationwide survey of 1000 randomly selected homes, the median magnetic field level away from appliances was found to be 0.6 mG and levels exceeded 3 mG in 5% of homes (Za93). Residential

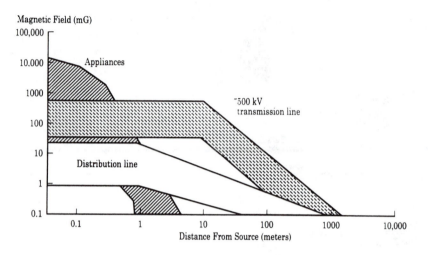

Figure 2.IV   Effect of Distance on Magnetic Field Levels For Various Sources
(Source: EPRI)

fields arising from power lines exceeded 1.0 mG in 20% of homes, 2.5
mG in 4.4% of homes, and 5 mG in 0.6% of homes.

The Effect of Distance on Magnetic Fields

It was noted earlier that field strengths decrease with distance from
the source of the field. The rate at which the field decreases, however,
depends on the nature of the source. With parallel conductors, such
as two electrical wires or conductors on power poles, fields decrease
more slowly with distance than the fields from appliances (Figure
2.IV). The principle is that magnetic fields decrease linearly with the
distance from single linear conductors but with the cube of the distance from circular conductors such as those in motors.

Another factor that determines the strength of the magnetic field
around parallel conductors such as those on power poles or in
household wiring is the distance between the two conductors. For
example, if you separate the two bonded electrical wires passing to
your electric lamp, you will find (if you are measuring the magnetic
field around those wires) that the magnetic field will increase as the
wires are separated.

One of the reasons that magnetic fields tend to be higher in older than in newer homes is that older wiring, known as "tube and knob," maintained several inches of separation between the two conductors. In newer homes, using cables in which the two conductors are bonded, magnetic field levels will tend to be lower.

Ground Currents

In addition to power lines, household wiring and appliances, an important source of magnetic fields in some homes is the "ground current" flowing through the plumbing system. As was noted above, the neutral conductor at the service box is connected to the water pipes below the house, which may, under certain circumstances, carry considerable return current. These currents, like all others, are a source of magnetic fields and may be an important source of exposure within the home. **Grounding** practices developed as a safety measure. Grounding to the plumbing system should not be disconnected as a means of reducing magnetic field exposures, since the hazard of electric shock will increase; however, research is being conducted to search for alternative grounding systems that will not reduce electrical safety.

Since the plumbing of neighboring homes is often connected, ground currents in one home may return to the utility system through the plumbing system of another home. For that reason, magnetic fields in any one home may reflect electricity use in neighbors' homes. In measuring the magnetic fields in your home, you may observe increasing field levels as your neighbors switch on appliances.

Harmonics

Still another fact about magnetic fields from electric power lines is that, although the utility generates power at 60 Hz, other frequencies may occur on utility lines. These are generally in multiples of 60, particularly 120 and 180 Hz. These other frequencies (harmonics) arise primarily as a result of the use of certain types of equipment by utility customers. Some have speculated that these harmonic frequencies could be important in producing biological effects, although there is no substantial evidence of this. Also, instruments vary in their ability to measure these **harmonics**. Should they be more carefully measured, or should they be ignored? Without knowing about their possible biological effects, we cannot answer that question at the present time.

Summary

In summary, we now have most of the basics that we need to consider exposures to individuals. The highlights are as follows:

- Power frequency electric fields, measured in V/m, can be shielded; the magnitude of these fields is related to voltage. The highest fields will generally be found around high-voltage transmission lines. Because voltage is relatively constant over time, the electric fields remain fairly constant at any one location.

- Magnetic fields, measured in Gauss or milligauss, cannot easily be shielded, and are related to current flow—the higher the current, the higher the magnetic field. Since current varies over time, as consumption of power varies, the magnetic fields vary substantially, but generally will be found in homes to be less than 1 milligauss away from appliances.

- The major sources of magnetic fields in homes are the neighboring power lines, household wiring, currents carried by the plumbing system to which the household wiring has been grounded, and appliances.

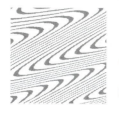

3

EMF Exposure Assessment

In this chapter, we move to the next stage of evaluating whether EMF produces effects to human health—the assessment of human exposure. As we shall see in subsequent chapters, assessment of exposure is critical to conducting epidemiologic studies (studies of health in human populations), and is a central concern in the evaluation of risks of EMF or any other agent suspected of producing human health effects; if epidemiologists cannot adequately assess exposure of the individual to a suspect agent, they cannot easily determine the influence of that agent on health or disease.

What does "exposure" mean? Whenever we make contact with an environmental factor (whether it be in the air, the drinking water, or our food) we are said to be "exposed" to that factor. For example, all of us are exposed to an atmosphere composed of about one–fifth oxygen, four–fifths nitrogen, and trace amounts of other gases. All of us are exposed to small amounts of chlorine placed intentionally in our drinking water supply, to sunlight and to food additives. Some of these may be beneficial, some may be harmful, some may be neither, and some may be both, depending on the level and duration of exposure.

Upon entering a space that contains an electric and/or a magnetic field, we become exposed to that field. Thus, for example, we are all continuously exposed to the earth's natural static (i.e., dc) magnetic field of about 500 milligauss, which in most situations has essentially the same strength indoors as it does outdoors.

What Is *Exposure Assessment* and Why Is It Important?

Exposure assessment is the determination or estimation of the magnitude and frequency of occurrence of exposure for an individual or group to an agent in the environment. It is useful to distinguish *exposure* from *dose*; exposure refers only to the measurement of the agent without particular regard (or knowledge of) those characteristics of the agent which are of significance to health, whereas dose refers to an assessment of that particular characteristic of exposure which is of significance to health. For the purposes of studying health effects in humans, investigators attempt the measurement of dose, but, in the absence of knowledge of the characteristics of exposure that are significant, they may have to measure exposure, using that as a rough measure of dose.

The measurement of exposure to ionizing radiation (e.g., from x–rays) may be illustrative. A film–badge exposure meter measures the exposure to an individual, but it is hardly a precise measure of dose. We know that the rate at which the exposure occurs is important (the film badge does not tell us that). We also know that the extent of the exposure to the body is important (the film badge does not tell us whether the exposure was limited to the area of the film badge or involved the entire body). Because both of these factors (as well as others) are important to estimating dose (and possible harm) we must have knowledge of the characteristics of exposure that are significant, and measurements of those characteristics of the exposure; the total exposure does not tell us that. As we shall see later, we have means of estimating exposures to EMF, but cannot measure dose.

The laboratory scientist studying the effects of exposure to an environmental agent has considerable advantage over the epidemiologist. Consider the situation where test animals are fed or otherwise exposed to a substance—call it factor "X." When evaluating the results of the experiment, the researcher knows precisely how much of factor "X" each animal received, and for how long exposure to "X" persisted. The researcher knows because he or she controls that exposure. Consequently, the researcher can chart the biological outcome against the precise amount of exposure to "X."

In studying people, the situation is usually far more difficult and far less precise. As individuals, we each maintain a unique, complex, and constantly changing lifestyle. For some agents, one can assess both current and past exposures simply by asking members of the study population. For example, in studies of the health effects of cigarette smoking, one can ask the individual about his or her current and past smoking habits. The method is not without problems—memories are fallible, or the individual may prefer to conceal the use of certain materials such as drugs, alcohol, or tobacco. Indeed sometimes people may be concealing their own behavior from themselves.

Nevertheless, the possibility of interviewing individuals about past behavior (e.g., cigarette smoking, breast feeding of infants) makes an epidemiological study easier to conduct than those inquiring into exposure to agents such as EMF where the individual has little personal knowledge of past exposure. This often leads to the use of **surrogates** for exposure; for EMF, for example, the title of the subject's job has often been used as a surrogate for occupational EMF exposure, and the proximity of a home to a power line has been used as a surrogate for personal exposure within the home.

To complicate matters for the epidemiologist interested in such chronic diseases as cancer, interest is not in current exposures, but to those which may have occurred before the onset of the disease. A surrogate for past EMF exposure that has been widely used is present EMF exposure, based on the assumption that exposures have been relatively constant over time, or at least, that the relative ranking of individual exposures has not changed, i.e., the persons with the highest exposures today were probably the same as those with the highest exposures previously.

Measurement of Fields (Br93a)

Two kinds of magnetic field measurements are often described in the literature—area measurements and personal exposure measurements. Area measurements are those taken in a specific area (as opposed to those to a given person); these provide information on levels within a space such as a home or school. While area measurements provide information on exposure levels in a particular location, they are imprecise measures of exposure to persons inhabiting or working in such a space, since exposure levels almost invariably vary within a space, therefore, they may not be reliable in assessing the exposure of a person moving within that space. For example, measurements taken within a kitchen are not reliable surrogates for the exposure of a person using that kitchen; we would need to know how much time the person spent in each location within the kitchen, particularly near appliances or other important sources of exposure.

Personal exposure measurements are meant to estimate the exposure patterns of individuals as they move from one environment to another.

For purposes of assessing personal EMF exposures, instruments have been developed that are compact, battery operated, and easy to wear on a belt or carry in a pocket. These may integrate exposure over the time worn (an ionizing radiation film badge is an example), or they may incorporate a computer that records and stores exposure information at frequent intervals. An example of the former is A-MEX (for Average Magnetic Field Exposure), which is worn like a wristwatch or in a pocket. It contains electronic circuitry that produces a cumulative record of the magnetic field exposure of the person wearing it. After a measurement session, the average magnetic field exposure during the period of measurement can be readily determined.

A more complex device, worn at the waist, is called the EMDEX (Electric and Magnetic Digital Exposure Meter). This device contains electronics that record a complete time–history of the magnetic field exposure for the period over which it is worn. An example of an exposure record obtained with such an instrument is shown in Figure 3.I, a record of an eight–year–old girl who wore an instrument on her belt during a typical school day, beginning in the afternoon upon returning home from school, and continuing through the night and next day.

Several interesting features can be noted in this record. First of all, note the variation that occurs as the child moves through the rooms of the house (3:30 p.m. —10:00 p.m.), each room of which may have somewhat different field levels. The higher exposures seen in the middle of the record result from her use of an electric blanket. During the next day, when she goes to school, a number of spikes or peaks are seen as she walks near power lines or appliances.

Typical indoor field levels were described in Chapter 2. Personal exposure levels are higher than those recorded with area measurements, since the latter are usually made in the center of rooms, away

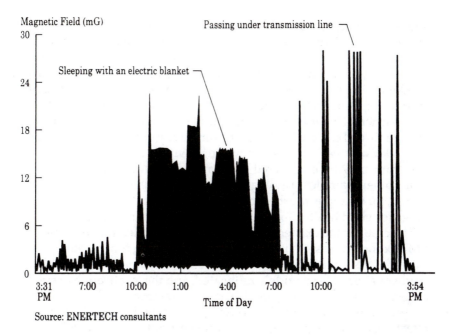

Figure 3. I   Magnetic Field Exposure Levels for an 8–Year–Old Girl

from appliances, whereas individuals who move freely about a residence will also record the exposures from appliances.

What Should We Measure—The Question of *Dose*

Ambient magnetic fields vary in both frequency and intensity. Understanding which pattern of exposure may be biologically effective could be very important in interpreting past results of epidemiological studies and in designing better studies. Are some frequencies more effective (or harmful) than others? Could there be thresholds, i.e., levels of exposure below which there is no effect, or could there be "windows," bands of exposure levels that produce biological responses, but below or above which there is little or no effect? These are questions directed to the issue of "dose"—those characteristics of the field (exposure parameters) that are most likely to produce biological effects.

Most toxicologists assume that high levels are more biologically harmful than are low levels. Most people almost automatically assume that this is true for EMF, i.e., that higher average exposure levels are potentially more harmful than lower exposure levels. However, some scientists have suggested that EMF may behave differently in this regard than other known agents. For example, Carl Blackman interprets his own research as showing the existence of "windows," certain frequencies or intensities of magnetic fields that are particularly important in explaining observed biological changes in cell cultures (Bl90a). The sensitivity of the retina of the eye to a relatively narrow frequency range within the electromagnetic spectrum may be considered an example of a biological window. Many other examples of biological windows occur; levels of most hormones, for example, must be maintained in the body within a narrow range for good health. Too much is bad, too little is bad.

The case for the existence of biologically significant windows for EMF exposures rests primarily on data regarding the movement of calcium ions towards or away from cell membranes (Bl90a). These studies have not been widely replicated, and the implication of such observations for defining an EMF dose is unclear.

Still another parameter that could be important in determining the effectiveness of exposure is an **intermittent**, as opposed to a constant, exposure. One set of observations that supports such an hypothesis is the work of Charles Graham. Graham has found that slowing of the pulse rate of human volunteers is more marked when the exposures are interrupted at 15–minute intervals; could this reaction to EMF be equivalent to reactions to many other stimuli, for which the organism can adapt to chronic, but not intermittent, exposures?

Intermittent exposures to humans are often more harmful then those that are continuing as can be illustrated with many known examples: alcoholic beverages consumed daily in moderation have been widely shown to have beneficial effects on health, whereas the same total quantity drunk on a single Saturday night (binge drinking, or "transients") can be harmful or even fatal.

To pursue this matter a bit further, consider the following example: suppose we wanted to study the effect of climate, and especially, temperature, on the incidence of heart attacks in American cities. What aspect of temperature should we measure? Should we study the average yearly temperature, or the maximum or minimum temperatures achieved during the year, or should we measure the number of days over 100 degrees or some other threshold level? Should we incorporate other factors into the exposure assessment? Temperature alone may not be as highly predictive of heart attacks as some combined measure of temperature and humidity.

While not a perfect analogy, this example of climate measurement and heart attack is not very different from those of EMF studies; in both cases, we are not sure exactly what to measure. In some ways, the heart attack problem is an easier one, since it is likely that it is the temperature on the day (or days) of the heart attack that is important, whereas with EMF and cancer, we suspect that it is the past exposure some years prior to diagnosis that is important.

Determining the appropriate magnetic field exposure parameters for individuals or groups under investigation poses an extremely knotty problem: which parameter of the complex magnetic field environment should we measure? What about rapidly occurring spikes or "**transients?**" Some scientists think that these transients could be important biologically. In assessing the individual's cumulative exposure over time periods such as days, weeks, or years, is it appropriate to take the average value of those cumulative exposures, or should we assume that only exposures above a certain "threshold value" are important?

In the absence of better knowledge of the most appropriate metric, scientists generally choose what is called the "**time–weighted average**," or TWA, and that is what they have often done in the epidemiological studies of EMF. In studies of childhood cancer and EMF exposure in which measurements of fields have been taken, investigators have often focused on a single daily area measurement that they assume is representative of past exposure.

If there are errors in our measurements of EMF exposure in epidemiological studies, the consequence may be that we will underestimate the risk of exposure. This is because poor exposure assessment does not allow us to accurately distinguish those who are highly exposed from those whose exposure is small. To illustrate: if we did not know which cigarette smokers smoked heavily and which smoked little, we would likely underestimate the risk of heavy smoking.

EMF Exposure Assessment in Epidemiology

Magnetic field levels within a home or workplace change over the course of the day, season, and year. For example, in a community with high summer heat and a high air-conditioning load, magnetic fields may well be higher in the summer than in the winter. What we really want to know about exposure in cancer epidemiologic study is not what the exposure to the study population is today, but rather what it was during previous years when disease may have first been initiated. Recreating those past exposures is what Professor Howard Wachtel, a neurophysiologist at the University of Colorado, has referred to as "magnetic field archeology," i.e., recreating the past from scraps of information that still exist.

A recently completed study obtained repeat measurements in the same residences that had previously been measured some years earlier. This study, conducted in Denver, shows a rather high degree of stability over time. Returning later to homes where measurements had been made in 1985, the investigators found a strong relationship between two sets of measurements made five years apart (Do93). This finding would suggest that current measurements are a fairly good surrogate for past exposure levels, but we need much more information on this point.

Another problem for the epidemiologist studying EMF is that all of us in modern society are exposed. Unlike other environmental agents, for which comparisons can be made of disease frequency in exposed and unexposed populations, with EMF we are *all* exposed; the question then becomes "who are the more-highly exposed, and who are less exposed?"

Occupational Exposures—Job Titles

A large number of epidemiological studies of persons engaged in electrical occupations have been conducted because of the assumption that such persons are exposed to higher levels of EMF. In many of these studies, a commonly used EMF exposure surrogate has been simply the kind of job one has—the **job title**. The epidemiologist makes the assumption that the type of work done by the individual is a reasonable basis on which to estimate that person's exposure to EMF. Of course, this is likely to be a very crude surrogate for exposure, since not all persons with the same job title experience the same exposure. For example, an electrician installing new equipment will usually experience very different exposures than an electrician working around operating machinery. Furthermore, work practices and equipment often change over time. A welder, for example, may change his equipment over the years, so that today's exposures may be very different from those encountered with previous equipment.

Then too, the use of job titles as a surrogate for exposure ignores the problem of possible confounders—other agents in the workplace, or lifestyle differences, that may influence disease incidence. Electricians or linemen in a study population may be different from other workers in many ways other than EMF exposure, and it is certainly possible, even likely, that these may contribute to differences in disease rates.

In more recent studies, actual measurements of EMF have replaced the use of job titles as a means of exposure assessment: these measurements show exposures in many electrical trades to be elevated, as will be described in chapter 10.

Spot Measurements

A surrogate of exposure used in some residential studies is the **spot measurement**. With this approach, researchers take the average of the EMF level in several rooms, making sure to steer clear of electrical appliances. The weakness of the spot measurement technique is that it captures information at only one instant in time—it is a snapshot and only a rough approximation of the long–term average EMF in that structure. It is somewhat like measuring the temperature at one moment in a room, and assuming that this represents the average temperature over long periods of time. Spot measurements of EMF often underestimate personal exposure, apparently because each of us spends time near appliances.

Distance to Power Lines as Exposure Surrogate

A simple surrogate of residential exposure is the distance between the home and the closest power line. This index assumes that the power line is the dominant source of exposure to persons in the home, an assumption that we know is frequently in error. It also ignores the amount of power being carried on the line, a key determinant of the magnetic fields surrounding that line.

A somewhat more sophisticated surrogate for classifying home exposures is the **wiring code**. In their 1979 study, Nancy Wertheimer and Ed Leeper introduced a wire coding scheme that classified homes in the Denver area according to both the estimated current–carrying capacity of the nearby power lines and the distance of the lines from the residence (Figure 3.II) (We79). The current version of this coding scheme

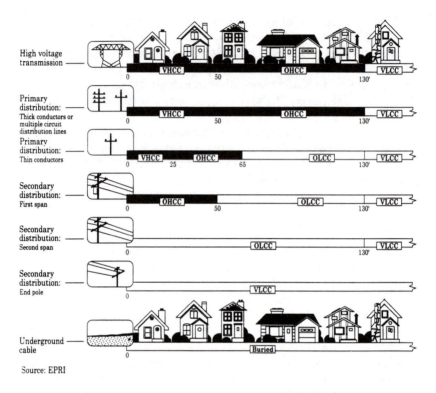

Source: EPRI

Figure 3.II Diagram For Determining Wire Code Configurations

classifies homes into very high (VHCC), ordinary high (OHCC), low (OLCC), very low (VLCC) and underground (UG) groups, representing assumed decreasing levels of residential exposure.

A further extension of the wire code concept is the recent use of a computer **model** based on the distance of the home to the line, the arrangement or configuration of the lines on the transmission line tower, and information about the power being carried on the line (Ah93b). This method has the advantage of using the actual loading on the line instead of estimated current–carrying capacity.

Summary

In summary, a variety of means for the assessment of exposure to EMF have been adopted., some for residential exposure, others for occupational exposure. This chapter has explored the nature of these methodologies, and their uses in conducting epidemiologic studies.

Two problems identified are our ignorance about the parameters of EMF exposure that are important to measure in assessing individual exposure, and, the difficulty of assessing exposures to the individual that may have occurred in the past, i.e., prior to the onset of disease.

III

HOW DOES IT
(EMF) WORK?

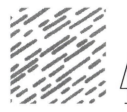

4

Mechanisms and Dose: How Does EMF Interact with Biological Systems?

When evidence of harm from exposure to an environmental agent is unequivocal, preventive measures are justified even when we have little understanding of "how it works." For example, epidemiologists believe that the evidence of an association between cigarette smoking and lung cancer is so overwhelming that it is not necessary to demand knowledge of biological mechanisms before undertaking a campaign to discourage smoking.

In the case of possible harm from EMF, however, many scientists consider the epidemiological evidence equivocal. Part of the reason that we cannot resolve the matter of EMF risk is that we do not know "how it works;" i.e., the mechanisms underlying the interaction of EMF with cells and tissues. If we are to design better epidemiological studies with which to resolve the issue of risk, we must do a better job of exposure assessment, and that will probably not happen until we can answer questions about mechanisms.

What Does *Mechanism* Mean?

Mechanism means different things to different people. The physicist wants to understand mechanisms at the atomic or molecular level—what are the physical means through which the electric and magnetic fields interact so as to produce changes in the function of the cell or tissue? To put this another way, how and where is the electric or magnetic field signal recognized by the cell? The biologist, on the other hand, wants to understand the mechanism through which the normal biochemical operation of the cell or tissue is altered. Biologically based mechanisms will be reviewed in Chapter 5.

The "Noise" Debate

Some skeptical scientists, particularly those from the physics community, are highly resistant to the notion of any biological effects from exposure to weak EMF ("weak" here refers to electric fields less than 300 V/m and magnetic fields less than 500 mG). They reason that the body is very active electrically, and that in the presence of so much physiological electrical activity, it is not plausible that cells could respond to an external EMF signal that is much smaller (by factors of thousands) than the body's internal electrical "noise."

The noise analogy is apt; in the same way that it is difficult to hear a conversation at a noisy party, the cell may not be able to "hear" a weak 60-Hz electrical message, given the chaotic electrical noise arising from the spontaneous electrical activity within the body. A leading skeptic and critic of most postulated theories of EMF effects is Robert Adair, Sterling professor of physics at Yale (and, incidentally, an expert on the physics of the game of baseball). He has written, "Any biological effects of weak ELF (extremely low frequency) fields on the cellular level must be found outside of the scope of conventional physics "(Ad 91). Others in the physics community share Adair's views (Be94, APS 95)

Analogies such as the noise analogy can take us only so far. While it is difficult to hear one conversation in a room buzzing with many, a listener can detect a violin even in concert with many other instruments. To the cell, is the 60-Hz EMF signal like a voice buried among the many at a noisy cocktail party or like a violin in an orchestra?

Some biologists and physiologists cite evidence that EMF can influence the metabolism of cells despite the random background electrical noise. For example, Kenneth McLeod, a biophysicist at the State University of New York at Stony Brook, has convincingly shown that chronically administered electrical currents can halt the loss of bone associated with osteoporosis, or hasten the growth of bone (McL92). However, field strengths necessary to produce such effects are far higher than ambient fields that have been alleged to produce human health effects.

Then, too, there is the story of the shark. Sharks and rays utilize an exquisitely sensitive organ (known as the Ampula of Lorenzini) to detect the electric fields generated by prey (Ka82). Apparently, the sharks and rays can respond to the electric field generated by the heart beat of the prey, even when the prey is buried in the bottom sand. The fields to which they are responding are extremely small (about 500 nanovolts/meter), providing strong evidence that at least some organisms can respond to field strengths even lower than the ambient 60-Hz fields found commonly in our residential environments. However, no highly electrically-sensitive organ systems such as the Ampula of Lorenzini are known to exist in any mammal, including man.

Whether our bodies can detect and respond to weak fields is one thing—harm is another. As Adair has pointed out, to perceive the light from a distant star is hardly reason to conclude that star-gazing is harmful.

Explanatory Theories

Four theories of EMF interaction that are now the subject of investigation are as follows:

Induced Currents.   Moving magnetic fields induce electrical currents in any conducting materials, whether they be wires of an electrical generator or tissues of the body. It can be argued that the mechanism that most plausibly explains the biological effects of EMF is the induction of electrical currents within tissues. To shed some light on this postulated mechanism, two kinds of calculations have been conducted. In one case, the induced currents are compared with those that occur naturally as a result of the body's electrical activities. In the other case, one compares the magnitude of induced currents with those known to produce observable effects in tissues. Let us examine each of these.

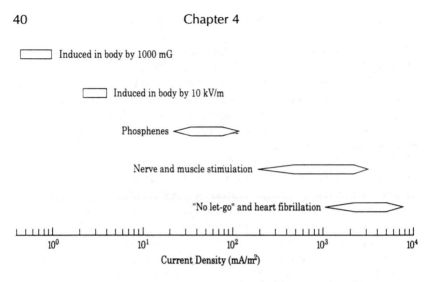

Figure 4.I   Approximate Current Density Thresholds For Various Responses

While we cannot easily measure currents around cells, it is possible to calculate the magnitude of currents that would be induced in tissues by ambient magnetic fields from conventional electrical sources, and to compare these with the currents that occur as a result of the body's own electrical activity. The result of such calculations shows that the induced currents are only a small fraction of those that occur normally, i.e., far less than 1%. It is this observation more than any other that leads some skeptics to dismiss the possibility that ambient power-frequency EMF can produce biological effects.

One can also compare the *calculated* current densities induced by ambient EMF with those necessary to produce observable effects in tissues. These are shown in Figure 4.1 The tapered ends of the density estimates for each response represent differences in sensitivity among individuals as well as uncertainty in converting the measured parameter to current density.

Note that known effects, such as the perception of flashes of light (phosphenes), or nerve and muscle fibrillation, require current densities of many tens to many thousands of milliamps per square meter, while the level of current density induced by 1 G magnetic field or a 10 kV/m electric field is about one milliamp per square meter.

For these reasons, many scientists do not believe that induced currents from power sources are of sufficient magnitude to produce biological effects. If this is correct, and if it is true that effects of EMF exposures can be demonstrated in the laboratory, then there *must be* a physical explanation of EMF effects other than induced currents.

Transients. This theory is really a variant of the induced-current theory just described. One way around the objection that induced currents are too low to produce effects is the notion that it may be *sudden* changes in magnetic fields (transients) that are responsible for biological effects.

When transients occur, the induced currents, which are proportional to the rate of change of the magnetic field, can change precipitously, though briefly, to levels that exceed those normally associated with the body's own physiological activity. This could provide an electrical signal that could be heard above the noise.

In part, transients have attracted a good deal of attention in the research community due to the work of Russell Reiter of the University of Texas, which appears to show that abrupt rises in magnetic fields are more likely to produce biological effects than slow increases in the magnetic field. Reiter has shown that exposing the pineal glands of rats to rapidly changing magnetic fields is more effective in suppressing melatonin secretion than exposures to slowly varying fields (Le91b). This can be explained in terms of induced currents that are operating to produce these biological effects.

How prevalent are electrical transients in our environment? Although research is only now pinpointing where and how often transients occur, there is already evidence that they may occur frequently, i.e., several times per day in the residential environment.

Resonance. Another group of theories of EMF interaction assumes that the 60-Hz EMF signal creates a **resonance** condition on the surface of the cell. Abraham Liboff, a physicist at Oakland University in Michigan, is a primary advocate of one such theory, which maintains that effects such as those employed in the cyclotron (where static or non oscillating fields combine with oscillating fields at specific frequency to accelerate the speed of a moving atomic particle) may operate in biological tissues (Li90). Liboff's theory is that applied fields and the earth's static field may combine to accelerate the movement of ions such as calcium though the cell membrane. His theory is based on observations in microscopic laboratory organisms that appear to become more motile only under resonance conditions between a static field and a **sinusoidal** field of particular frequency. Other scientists have been unable to duplicate these findings and serious theoretical limitations in the resonance theory have also been noted (Ad91).

Direct Magnetic Field Effects. Another theory that might explain how cells "sense" EMF involves the means utilized for navigation by some bacteria, birds, honeybees, fish, and salamanders. These animals all contain tiny bits of a mineral, known as magnetite, that actually constitute small magnets that can be moved by ambient magnetic fields. Joseph Kirschvink, at California Institute of Technology, has studied these materials for years, and suspects that they might be the means through which certain EMF-induced biological effects are produced in tissues.

Kirschvink has trained bees to detect static magnetic fields to locate a source of sugar. Using this test system, he has been able to examine whether bees can also respond to power-frequency fields. It seems that they can, but they are far less sensitive to 60-Hz fields than they are to static fields. While the bee can detect and respond to 3-mG static fields, it cannot detect power-frequency fields below about 3 G.

But do humans have magnetite in their bodies? Kirschvink has found some evidence of magnetite in human brain tissue, but we do not know if magnetite has any function in humans at all; like the appendix, it may simply be present as a vestige. Further, Kirschvink's calculations would appear to show that if these magnetite receptors could respond to ac fields at all, the field intensities would have to be much higher than those we normally encounter in the environment.

EMF in Bone Healing

One has to be in awe of the ability of the human body to heal itself when injured. The vast majority of bone fractures heal themselves, if the bone is held in a reasonably normal and stable position. Occasionally, even when well-positioned, a fracture will fail to heal, a so-called "non-union." This condition can be nasty, limiting the return to useful function and predisposing the patient to infection and disability. It is for these fractures that electric currents have been used to stimulate healing.

It has long been known that bone has the characteristic of being "piezoelectric." That is, when put under stress, as in walking, the stressed bone generates an electrical current. Some years ago, Andrew Bassett suggested that these normally occurring electrical currents are necessary to the maintenance of normal bone, and that fractured bones may fail to heal because with the bone immobilized the piezoelectric currents are not activated (Ba92). As a consequence, he induced electrical currents in the fracture site using an external stimulating device and found that bone healing was accelerated. Many investigators worldwide have since reported this technique to be successful. This phenomenon convinces many people that applied electrical currents can produce biological effects, especially in light of the demonstration by McLeod that sinusoidal 60-Hz fields are effective in initiating bone growth, albeit at field strengths far higher than those normally associated with the power line environment (McL92).

While the McLeod results are impressive, we still do not know just how the mechanism works, that is, how EMF heals bones. And certainly, the ability of EMF to promote healing in bones provides no evidence that EMF causes cancer or any other health effect. What it does do is to demonstrate that some tissues can respond to electric currents.

Where Is the Message Heard?

One issue that occupies scientists is the identification of the *site* at which the interaction with EMF might occur. Is the EMF message "heard" at the cell membrane, the cell nucleus, or elsewhere (possibly at the junction between cells)?

A leading candidate for the site of interaction is the cell membrane. The reason that attention quite naturally focuses on this delicate covering of the cell is that an externally induced field does not easily penetrate the cell membrane. Further, it is at the cell membrane that the cell normally receives its command and control messages from other cells and organs in the body; the membrane is the switchboard or nerve center of the cell.

It should not be assumed that *all* of the body's cells are equally sensitive to EMF; it may be that only certain cells are adapted to sense ambient EMF. In the next chapter, the melatonin hypothesis will be discussed. That hypothesis suggests that effects of fields may be sensed through the pineal gland. If this is the case, then where is the message heard? A possible receptor organ is the retina of the eye, the thin layer of light-sensitive cells at the back of the eye, which we know responds to electromagnetic energy in the form of light. It is possible that the retina is also sensitive to power-frequency EMF. On the other hand, EMF may be detected in any part of the neural pathway from retina to pineal gland—we just don't know (Ol90).

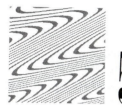

5

EMF in the Laboratory

Laboratory investigation can contribute to risk assessment in two ways: first, if disease can be produced in animals exposed to a specific agent, particularly at levels of exposure that approximate those found in the human environment, this strengthens the case for that agent as a toxic agent. Second, if laboratory studies of simple cellular systems can provide evidence of just where and how that agent produces biological effects, then such information can help us design better epidemiological studies to resolve the question of effects in human populations.

The Normal Cell

A living cell is essentially a liquid-filled bag, contained by a membrane (the "bag") and whose operation is controlled by the genetic mechanism located within a central compartment, the cell nucleus. The cell membrane is not simply a rudimentary barrier, but is a highly sophisticated organ in itself. The chemical composition inside the cell differs considerably from that outside the cell, and the cell membrane is required to perform highly selective functions in maintaining these differences—it is a gatekeeper as well as a gate. It is also a highly specialized receptor for chemical messengers, such as hormones, that can alter the function of the cell. As we shall see, the membrane is important in the consideration of potential EMF health effects since it is a possible target for the interaction of EMF with the human body.

The genes of each human cell contain information for the synthesis of as many as 100,000 proteins. Not all are required for the function of each cell or organ system; therefore, the majority of these genes are "switched off" most of the time. Furthermore, many functions may need to be enhanced or suppressed as conditions require. For example, the need for higher concentrations of pregnancy hormones will be mediated through an up-regulation of the genes responsible for that synthesis. How does the cell control these various processes? Messages are received from outside the cell through means of chemical agents, which impinge on and interact with the cell membrane. These messages are then transmitted through the membrane to the interior of the cell, where other secondary messengers regulate individual gene functions. The nervous system. operating in a fashion similar to a telephone long-distance system, provides another means of signaling to tissues.

Just as cells have a long-distance telephone system, they can also chat with neighbors across the back fence. There is recent evidence that in addition to receiving signals from more-distant parts of the body, cells are able to communicate adjacent cells through channels called gap junctions, through which some chemicals can pass. Although the function of these channels is not yet entirely clear, they too have been suggested as a possible site of EMF interactions with cells.

Cancer, Mutation, and Carcinogenesis

The cancer process probably begins with permanent damage to the genetic mechanism of a cell (**mutagenesis**), producing what is known as **initiation**. Following initiation, the genetically altered cell may remain dormant for months or years until some stimulus causes

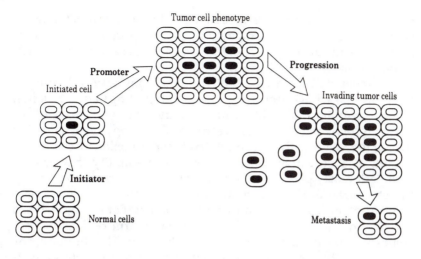

Figure 5.1   Stages in the Evolution of a Cancer (Pi93)

the cell to begin proliferating, thus beginning the second step of the cancer process, known as **promotion**. Only then does the inability of the cell to control growth become apparent.

Cancer Promotion and Promoters

Promotion denotes the stimulation of the initiated cell to grow into a mass, known as a **tumor**, but one that still does not have malignant characteristics. Small tumors in the bowel (polyps) are thought to be examples of promoted but not yet malignant tumors. In contrast with initiation, promotion is a reversible process, as shown in Figure 5.1 For example, in some experimental systems in the laboratory, tumors subjected to promotion for a short period of time will show growth, but then regress when the promoter is removed.

How important is promotion, compared with initiation, in the development of human cancers? Henry Pitot, professor of Oncology and Pathology at the University of Wisconsin, believes that understanding promotion is the key to understanding human cancer. He says, "Initiation, which appears to be an extremely ubiquitous phenomenon, is almost a given in the natural development of neoplasia in the human. However, unless the stage of promotion intervenes either exogenously or endogenously, such "spontaneously" initiated cells will never produce disease in the individual. It is actually the stage of promotion that is probably the most important in our understanding of the development of human neoplasia and the risk of environmental chemicals." (Pi93)

A number of observations, both from the laboratory and from human pathology, have been interpreted as suggesting that stimulation of tissue proliferation is likely to accelerate or promote cancer. For example, following partial surgical removal, the rapidly regenerating liver of the rat is highly susceptible to cancer induction by chemicals.

Clinical observations also support the possibility that growth stimulation may play a role in the development of cancer. Anything that stimulates tissue growth, such as in tissue repair of injuries (scar formation), may promote cancer development. For example, it is a practice in northern parts of India to stay warm by keeping hot stones in a pouch against the skin of the abdomen. The chronic burns produced in the skin by the constant heat irritation frequently develop skin cancers.

The situation appears to be complicated; as with everything related to cancer formation, simplistic conclusions are often wrong. For example, there are also many conditions under which cells rapidly proliferate that do not lead to cancer. Growth of the fetus to adulthood requires many trillions of cell divisions; why do we not all have cancer? Another example: the lining cells of the small intestine are rapidly and persistently proliferating, yet cancers of the small intestine are rare.

Still, there is good evidence that some known human carcinogens do act through their ability to stimulate proliferation of cells. Two examples are asbestos and hormones such as the estrogens.

Cancer Progression

The third stage of the cancer process, **progression**, requires still another stimulus. The proliferated cell mass begins spreading (metastasizing) elsewhere in the body. Even this three-step model may be overly simplistic; the development of bowel cancer is now thought to require at least eight discrete mutations.

Mutagenic agents are not limited to industrial chemicals or ionizing radiation. Many common foods contain chemicals that have been shown to be mutagenic. These include pepper, cinnamon, and heated, browned, or charred foods such as toast or charcoal-broiled hamburgers. In addition, agents produced within the body itself, such as hormones, can produce mutations. Viruses can also cause cancer, possibly through their ability to insert themselves into genes of the host cell.

Although only agents that produce mutations can initiate the cancer process, certain non-mutagenic agents can serve as promoters. While initiating agents are thought to be active even at very low levels, without a threshold or lower limit of effect, promoting agents are believed to cause effects only above a threshold level of exposure.

Does EMF Play a Role in Cancer?

With this brief survey of cancer biology as background, let us look at laboratory investigations of EMF as a possible carcinogen. We will examine the following questions:

- Is EMF an initiating agent, i.e., mutagenic?

- Is EMF a cancer promoter—as examined in living animals?

- Is EMF a cancer promoter—as examined in isolated cells?

- Does EMF stimulate cancer progression?

- Could EMF impair the immune response?

- Does EMF impair melatonin production?

Is EMF Mutagenic?

The scientific literature contains more than 50 reports of studies on possible genotoxic (harmful to genes) effects of EMF exposure. Many of these are studies of isolated cells exposed to EMF in the laboratory, while others are studies of mutagenesis in living animals following such exposures. A great range of exposure conditions is represented in these studies, and a variety of techniques are applied. While a few of the studies are reported by the investigator as showing positive effects, the great preponderance of evidence leads to the conclusion that there are no reproducible mutagenic or genotoxic effects of electric or magnetic field exposures (McC93a, Mu93). It is for this reason—the failure of EMF to produce mutations— that investigation of EMF has shifted from the initiation stage to later stages in the process of carcinogenesis.

Studies of EMF Cancer Promotion—in Whole Animals

The laboratory model often used to test the possibility of cancer promotion involves the skin of the mouse. In a typical experiment, the skin of the mouse is first treated with a known chemical initiator. One such treatment does not normally cause skin cancer, but if application of the initiating agent is followed by repeated treatments with a known promoter, cancers will almost always occur. Without the prior treatment with the initiator, the promoting agents alone do not produce cancer. In this model, both exposures are necessary.

A study of this design, using magnetic field exposure as a possible promoter, was carried out by Maria Stuchly and colleagues at Health and Welfare Canada. When mouse skin was first treated with a chemical initiator (dimethylbenzanthracene) and then exposed to magnetic fields, there was no increase in skin tumors, suggesting that magnetic fields alone are not a promoting agent (St92b). However, when the magnetic fields were applied together with the commonly used promoters, phorbol esters, the number of skin tumors was increased beyond that found with phorbol esters alone. This outcome is interpreted as showing the effect of a *copromoter*, an agent that enhances the effect of another cancer promoter, but that by itself is not sufficient to produce an effect. These experiments are difficult to do and difficult to interpret; indeed, the same laboratory has reported that they have been unable to replicate the earlier finding (McL93).

In a Swedish study headed by Agneta Rannug, investigators have used a liver model instead of a skin model. In this research, the mice were treated with an initiating agent (diethylnitrosamine) and a promoting agent (phenobarbital), as well as with magnetic fields. Rather than an effect suggesting an increase in cancer formation, there was a suggestion that the magnetic fields reduced the effect of the cancer-causing chemicals (Ra93).

In contrast, another study found apparent evidence of a promoting effect, this time on mammary tumors in rats. At the Oncology Research Center in Tbilisi, Georgia, Dzhemal Beniashvili and his colleagues first exposed rats to a chemical known to initiate mammary tumors and then to either static or variable (50-Hz) magnetic fields of 200 mG. They found that magnetic fields both accelerated the appearance of tumors and increased the number of animals with tumors (Be91). The effects of ac exposures were greater than those of static exposures. An increase in mammary cancer in rats exposed to EMF has also been found by German investigators (Me93).

What is the explanation for these apparently conflicting results? One possibility is that all the results are correct and meaningful; that magnetic fields cause different effects under different circumstances, sometimes promoting cancer, sometimes protecting against cancer. There may be other explanations as well, explanations related to differences in exposure conditions, diet, or any other experimental variable. Finally, it is possible that there are no effects—the positive studies are due to chance or bias. We just don't know.

Nor do we understand the precise applicability of these laboratory models to human health. The models are very sensitive to the order in which drugs are applied, the timing of the exposures, and even the diet of the animals; changes in any of these can affect the outcome. While these experiments can be useful in helping us to understand how EMF could affect cancer processes, they need to be done carefully – often they cannot be repeated by other scientists—but ultimately, they may provide the biological understanding that we need to design better epidemiological studies.

Lifetime Studies in Animals

Over the past 30 years, the "gold standard" for testing an agent suspected of being carcinogenic is the study of laboratory animals exposed to the agent throughout their lifetimes.

Four laboratories have initiated studies of animals exposed to magnetic fields throughout their lifetimes: two are in the United States, one is in Canada, and the other is in Sweden.

Three of these studies differ from the conventional protocol for animal studies. They are specifically designed to test EMF as a promoter of cancer. To test this hypothesis, investigators are first exposing animals to a known carcinogen (such as ionizing radiation or carcinogenic chemicals) and then following this initiating exposure with lifelong exposures to magnetic fields. The exposures are many times higher than those generally occurring in the everyday environment. The fourth study, conducted by the National Institutes of Environmental Health Sciences, does not involve the use of an initiating agent, but examines magnetic fields alone.

Table 5.1: Reported Cellular Changes in Cells Exposed
to EMF in The Laboratory

Gene expression; (Go93b)
Calcium metabolism; (Wa92a)
Immune function (Wa92a)
Neural cell stimulation; (O'C88)
Electroreception (Ka82)
Cellular copromotion; (Ca93a)
Diatom motility; (Li90)
Cell-to-cell communication (proposed, unpublished)

The results of these studies, likely to be available in the next few years, are likely to have a strong influence on the scientific judgment of the possible carcinogenicity of EMF.

Studies of EMF Effects in Cells

Many studies of EMF exposure on isolated cells have been conducted in order to examine just how EMF may influence cellular physiology. Subjects of these studies include the suppression of melatonin synthesis (discussed later in this chapter), interference with immunity, and certain gene functions that might alter our ability to control tumor growth (Table 5.1). Many or most of these studies have been conducted with magnetic field strengths considerably higher than those typically found in the home or workplace.

Studies of possible cancer promotion can be carried out in isolated cells of a strain that responds to tumor-promoting agents by acquiring malignant characteristics. These have sometimes been interpreted as showing promoting effects of EMF exposure, while other studies in the same laboratory have shown just the opposite—magnetic fields suppress promotion (Ca93a, Ca93b).

Calcium is important physiologically as a "messenger;" that is, many cell functions are known to be triggered by alterations in calcium release or uptake by the cell membrane. Studies of EMF exposure and altered calcium metabolism are inconsistent. Some studies show increased uptake by cells, while others show increased release of calcium.

Another direction of laboratory study with EMF involves the processes known as transcription and translation, i.e., the processes by which the genes within the nucleus send messages into cell fluids that control the essential processes of cell metabolism. Reba Goodman and Ann Henderson, working at Columbia University and Hunter College, respectively, have found that under a variety of conditions, exposure to EMF can result in alteration of the translation/transcription process that increases protein synthesis (Go93b).

A number of factors are known to alter protein synthesis. While some of them may lead to potentially harmful effects, others are protective, so the observation of an effect on gene function alone does little to tell us whether EMF is damaging to human health. Further, not everyone has been able to observe the same changes that the New York investigators have found (Pa92, Sa93a). Whether this is the result of different exposure conditions or differences in the cell strain being examined is not clear.

Does EMF Stimulate Cancer Progression?

A number of laboratory systems have been developed to examine the ability of agents to stimulate the progression phase of cancer. These can be carried out either in isolated cells or in whole animals. Several of these studies have been performed with magnetic field exposure. For example, in one study, leukemic cells were implanted in mice that were then exposed to magnetic fields at different field strengths (ranging from 14 to 5000 mG) each day throughout the duration of the life span of the animals. There was no difference in the survival, spleen or body weights of the animals compared with those of unexposed animals (Th88). Other studies of progression in isolated cells as well as in whole animals have been conducted without any consistent findings.

Cancer and The Immune System

Mutation followed by promotion of the cancerous cell is only part of the explanation for the appearance of clinical cancer. It is quite clear that the body has defenses against the growth and spread of cancer, so that at least two processes must occur for the cancer cell to grow and become lethal: the cancer cell must be present and stimulated to grow, and the body's defenses must be overcome.

The immune system is complex, consisting of cells that circulate in the blood (white cells), proteins that also circulate (antibodies, cytokines), and solid organs (the thymus, lymph nodes, and spleen). The primary function of this system is to recognize and contain invaders of the body such as bacteria or foreign bodies (e.g. slivers, stings).

The immune system also functions to distinguish tumor cells from normal cells. It is well known that a defective immune system predisposes a person to cancer as well as to infection. For example, persons whose immunity is depressed because of genetic disease, drug suppression, stress, or exposure to ionizing radiation will be at increased risk of cancer.

James Morris of the Battelle Pacific Northwest Laboratory examined the effects of electric fields at various field strengths on the immune systems of mice and rats and found no effects (Mo83). Other investigators have studied the effects of electric fields on cultured lymphocytes and found a decrease in the function of these cells (Ly88). There has also been a report of decreased function of lymphocytes exposed to magnetic fields (Co83). There are no major studies of EMF and immunity in human populations.

The Melatonin Hypothesis

An intriguing set of observations suggesting a possible mechanism of cancer promotion by EMF is related to the suppression of melatonin, a hormone secreted by the pineal gland and thought to have a modifying effect on immunity and cancer development.

The pineal gland is a pea-size gland located at the base of the brain. Until recently, little was known about its function other than that it has something to do with reproduction. Tumors of the gland (pinealomas) are extremely rare, but when they occur among children, they produce precocious puberty, i.e., premature development of the genitalia and adult hair growth and distribution. Otherwise, the general view of the pineal gland in the past was that the gland is a useless vestige, something like the appendix.

The discovery of the hormone melatonin, secreted by the pineal gland, and the recognition of melatonin's role in reproduction and in maintaining daily biological rhythms, greatly accelerated interest in the pineal gland. It was also found that melatonin synthesis does not take place at constant rates, but occurs mostly at night; the hormone's production is suppressed by light, and its secretion is reduced if daylight hours are artificially extended. Thus the pineal gland became the prototype of a "neuroendocrine transducer," an organ that converts environmental signals (in this case, light) to hormone messengers.

Today, many additional functions are attributed to this tiny gland. Recent evidence suggests that the pineal gland not only controls certain sex hormones, but may also have a role in an organism's susceptibility to cancer. For example, animals that have had their pineal glands removed are more susceptible to induced cancer, while animals treated with melatonin are less susceptible to experimentally induced cancers (Bl90b).

Because the pineal gland responds to light, it was quite natural for investigators to speculate that other frequencies of the electromagnetic spectrum, such as power-frequency EMF, might also influence melatonin. There now exists a rather large literature detailing the responses of a variety of species (rats, hamsters, baboons, birds) to various EMF exposures, including electric, magnetic, and static fields. While effects (suppression of melatonin) are occasionally seen (for example, Ka93), no consistent, strong effects are seen (Br92b).

What could this inconsistency mean? Either EMF suppresses melatonin, but under conditions that we do not understand and cannot control, or that the observations of suppression are somehow flawed.

Because rodents are much more sensitive to suppression of melatonin by light than are humans, there is also a question of whether magnetic field suppression of melatonin in animals, if real, can be extrapolated to humans. Until recently, no systematic human experimental work had been conducted. Now there is a preliminary report of work on 33 human volunteers. The results appear to show that while not all humans show a decrease in melatonin levels with magnetic field exposures, some individuals do respond (Gr93). This work, being conducted by Charles Graham at the Midwest Research Institute in Kansas City, Missouri, is continuing.

The question of EMF as a suppresser of melatonin remains unresolved. Results in laboratory animals has been inconsistent, human observations are very limited, and the role of melatonin in cancer development remains highly speculative.

Summary

To support the assessment of the risk of EMF in human populations, there has been a very large effort in many scientific laboratories to

identify consistent biological effects of EMF exposure in the laboratory. The only established observation is the absence of a mutagenic
effect. While many cellular effects have been noted by one or sometimes two investigators, none has consistently been verified—many
either cannot be replicated or results have been inconsistent. The
confused state of affairs has led one scientist (H. B. Graves) to suggest a resemblance of this field of science to the Cheshire Cat of *Alice
in Wonderland*. You will remember that the cat would appear to Alice
unexpectedly in the oddest places, sometimes whole, sometimes
only the grin visible. Sometimes you see it . . . sometimes you don't.
Are such laboratory observations figments of the investigators'
imagination, a Cheshire cat, or are they real phenomena that we do
not understand well enough to specify the conditions under which
they occur?

IV

ASSESSING RISKS TO HEALTH

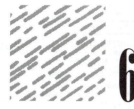

6
What is
Risk Assessment?

Human beings face a great number of risks from a variety of sources (Figure 6.I provides a partial listing).

Some risks, such as those arising from very rare events, are often ignored, while others, equally rare, get a great deal of our attention; lightening strikes are an example of the former, nuclear power plant accidents an example of the latter. Clearly there are objective as well as subjective factors involved in our evaluation of risks.

How do we make judgments about which risks are important and which are not? For some risks, such as automobile accidents, actuarial data are easily available—we know precisely how many deaths occur per year. For others, such as those that might arise from exposure to environmental agents in our air, water, or food, we are much less certain. The science of making judgments about the existence and magnitude of risks is called, logically, **risk assessment**.

What is the relevance of risk assessment to this book? First of all, the judgment of whether EMF is harmful to human health will be made on the basis of rules laid down for risk assessment in general. Therefore, the reader will need some perspective on how this process is conducted.

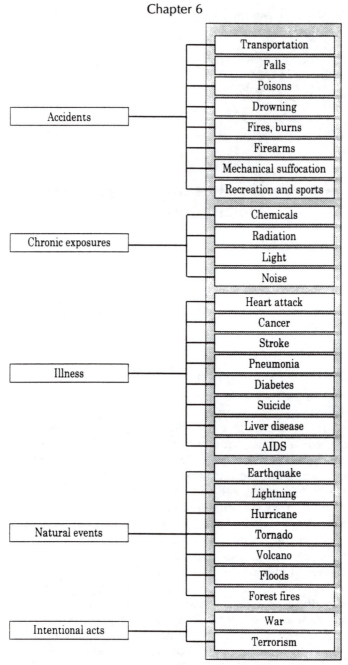

Figure 6.1   Examples of Human Risks

Second, although risk assessment practices are relied upon to set environmental policy, risk assessment is rather an arcane art, not widely taught or understood. The principles of risk assessment described here apply equally to risks from other factors, such as air pollution or dietary fat.

By convention, risk assessment involves the following four steps:

Hazard Identification: In this first stage of the process, where the risks of a new potentially toxic agent are still quite unknown, researchers attempt to ascertain the general nature of the effects that may be associated with exposure to this agent: is it a **carcinogen**? Does it affect reproduction or behavior? A variety of techniques may be used for this assessment, including epidemiology and laboratory studies.

Exposure-Response Assessment: Knowing that the agent is harmful, the next question to be answered is: how harmful, and under what conditions of exposure? This kind of information can be derived from studies of humans exposed at different levels, or from animal studies. An example: if persons smoking 20 cigarettes per day experience x number of lung cancers, what risk of lung cancers will occur among persons smoking 10 cigarettes per day? 40 cigarettes per day? Answers to these questions allow the construction of an exposure-response relationship.

Exposure Assessment: Once researchers know what kind of effects they are looking for, and the harm resulting from various levels of exposure, the next question to ask is: how frequently will this effect occur? Is esposure to this agent a public health problem, or does it occur so rarely that it can be dismissed or given a low priority? The answer depends upon the number of persons who are exposed to the agent, and the average level of exposure.

Risk Characterization: Given information on both risk and exposure, an estimate can now be made of the total number of cases that will be expected from this source of exposure – the risk characterization. An example may be useful. Suppose we are concerned with possible harm from human consumption of mercury contaminated fish. In order to estimate the public health impact of this source of exposure, we must know the following:

- What health effects are produced in humans by ingestion of mercury?

- What are the mercury contamination levels found in fish?

- Given these levels of exposure, what effects will be produced in people who eat fish?

- How many persons eat fish?

From the data collected in our hypothetical example, we are now in a position to make a statement such as, "given our knowledge of mercury toxicity and current dietary practices in the United States, it can be estimated that X number of cases of Y disease occur in the United States each year." Of course, such an estimate should also make explicit all of the assumptions and uncertainties that are inherent in such an estimate.

Risk Management: What then? The agency or officials responsible for public health must then make a judgment of whether this level of risk is acceptable, and what can reasonably be done to minimize those risks. This process is known as Risk Management. Risk management is not solely a scientific undertaking, but is a process that takes into account several factors, including the possible harm of alternatives, economic considerations, and inevitably, public perceptions of the risk that may be very different from the risk estimate derived from the process of risk assessment described above.

It has often noted that public concerns regarding certain risks may differ greatly from those of experts. A number of reasons for these discrepancies have been suggested; one of these is the degree of control that the individual has over the risk. For example, many people feel much safer in their cars than they do in airplanes, primarily because they feel a sense of control in their cars, whereas they have no control over the airplane in which they are flying.

Another reason is that people's judgment of the magnitude of risk is often determined by how often they read or hear about a particular risk. For this reason, studies show that most people, when asked about the relative frequency of suicide versus murder respond that murder is more common. In fact, suicide is 6 times more common than murder in the United States. The psychologist Paul Slovic finds that people's estimates of risks such as these are dependent, among other things, upon the frequency with which the risk is reported!

Changing Concepts of Risk

Are all exposures to toxic agents at any concentration harmful? Can chemical or physical agents be divided into those that are harmful and those that are harmless? More specifically, are there agents that can cause cancer at any level of exposure? Answers to these questions are key to our risk policies, and have undergone considerable change over past decades, but the questions are still not entirely resolved.

Prior to the 1960s, it was assumed that there was a threshold, or level of exposure below which no effects would be observed. This is a reasonable assumption and one all of us make in managing our daily lives. If a 200-mile-an-hour hurricane is known to knock down chimneys, we do not assume that a gentle breeze of, say, five miles an hour will knock down a small number of chimneys; we do assume a threshold. Similarly, although we accept that drinking a bottle of whiskey in one sitting has a certain probability of being lethal, we also accept that there is a reasonable level of consumption, let us say, one cocktail, that will not kill anyone (although it might be harmful to the unborn child of a pregnant woman). In the same way, it was once thought that there were safe levels of exposure to carcinogenic agents (such as ionizing radiation) that would not produce cancer.

In the 1960s, three lines of thinking were adopted that changed thinking on environmental risks of cancer and formed the basis of our modern environmental policy. They were: awareness of the role of mutations in cancer development, abandonment of the threshold model, and the strong suspicion of industrial pollutants as environmental mutagens, and therefore, carcinogens. Let us examine each of these.

Mutagens as Carcinogens.   In the 1960s, it was first recognized that damage to the genetic material in the cell is a first step in the process of initiating a cancer, therefore, any agent that is mutagenic also becomes a prospective carcinogen.

The Demise of Thresholds.   Following the Second World War, the notion of thresholds came under question. There was the recognition that safety is never absolute—some risk always exists, no matter how small the exposure. Someone *may* die from a single cocktail; somewhere a chimney *may* fall over with a five-mile-an-hour breeze.

The challenge to the threshold concept arose from the biological, and particularly, the radiological research community. The Nobel Prize-winning biologist, Herman Muller (1890–1960), in studying the genetic effects of ionizing radiation in fruit flies, had been unable to identify a threshold; it appeared to him that even very small exposures of radiation were capable of producing damage to genetic material.

Given those observations, the absence of a demonstrable threshold and the role of mutations in the cancer process, the notion of safe thresholds of exposure was abandoned in favor of a non-threshold model, which assumes that effects occur at low or even very low exposures *in proportion to* effects seen at high levels of exposure.

Another assumption widely adopted for the purposes of risk assessment is the so-called *linear* theory. This implies that effects will be found in the same proportion to exposure found at high exposure levels.

A hypothetical example will further illustrate the concept of linearity. Assume that a risk of cancer is observed among persons exposed to a substance found in the work environment at high concentrations, say 100 **parts per million**. The linear hypothesis states that persons exposed at much lower levels, 1 part per million, will have one hundredth the risk observed at high concentrations.

Industrial Pollutants as Environmental Mutagens. With the awakening interest in the environment, perhaps best dated to publication of Rachel Carson's *Silent Spring,* (Ca62) there arose concern that environmental pollution by chemicals, particularly pesticides, could have effects not only on the environment, but on human health as well. The idea that environmental contaminants were an important cause of cancer in human populations became fixed in public thinking.

Permissible (Acceptable) Levels of Risk

If the notion of a safe threshold is replaced by the concept of a risk at any level of exposure, then some arbitrary level of acceptable risk must be adopted. What levels of risk from environmental exposures, whether chemical or physical sources (such as radiation) are permitted by regulatory agencies?

One commonly adopted standard is that the additional risk posed by a particular chemical exposure or radiation source should not increase the risk of cancer by more than one in a million per lifetime of exposure. To put risks of this magnitude into perspective, if the risk of cancer in the general population were exactly 25%, then the permissible cancer rate in the exposed population should not rise above 25.000001%. Of course, such a small increase could never be detected or validated.

A one-in-a-million risk is difficult for most of us to visualize. Here are some examples of activities calculated to produce a risk of that magnitude—one-in-a-million risk of death:

- Traveling 1000 miles by train

- Traveling 30 miles by bus

- Bicycling for 5 miles

- Smoking 1.5 cigarettes

- Living in a brick house for 10 days (because of the additional exposure to the natural radioactivity in bricks)

- Drinking half a quart of wine

No Safe Levels **Becomes Law**

Congress was well aware of these developments in the evolving concepts of cancer causation. In 1958, under the sponsorship of Congressman James Delaney of New York, an amendment (the Delaney Amendment) to the Food, Drug, and Cosmetic Act was enacted. Delaney's wife had just died of cancer and the Congressman wanted to limit the exposure of the entire population to carcinogenic materials. On the basis of the new assumptions regarding environmental pollutants described above, the removal of industrial chemicals from the food supply became the keystone of cancer prevention policy. The Delaney Amendment stated that any substance that had been shown to cause cancer in laboratory animals, *at any concentration*, should be prohibited from the food supply. This is, of course, an even more rigid standard than one permitting exposures estimated to limit risks to one in a million per lifetime; it states that *no* cancer risk will be permitted. The Delaney Amendment remains on the books today.

Beginning in the 1960s, risk assessment emerged as a recognized discipline and an important tool for decision making. Formal procedures for performing animal bioassays were established in the 1960s and 1970s; and formal risk assessment began to be conducted regularly in the late 1970s. The Society for Risk Analysis, which now has approximately 1500 members, was created in 1980.

Among the U.S. governmental agencies that have adopted quantitative risk assessment are the Environmental Protection Agency, the Food and Drug Administration, and the Agency for Toxic Substances and Disease Registry.

Evidence for Estimating Risks

Risk assessment incorporates evidence from two main sources: studies of human populations exposed to the suspect agent and laboratory studies of animals exposed to the agent.

Epidemiology. Risk estimates based on observations of the species in which we are most interested, human subjects living under real life conditions, are by far the most reliable as the basis for risk assessment. Epidemiological data avoid the need for uncertain extrapolation from observations of laboratory animals, and sometimes from high exposures to low.

Use of Laboratory Animals. Frequently, adequate epidemiological evidence is not available, either because the chemical or pharmaceutical is new, or because exposures to human populations have not been sufficient to produce effects that might be detectable. Under these circumstances, risk assessment will be based on toxicological studies of laboratory animals to which large doses of a suspect chemical are fed daily throughout their lifetimes. Risks to humans from much smaller and less-frequent exposures are then calculated on the basis of mathematical models.

Extrapolating From Animal Studies and High Doses to Humans and Low Doses: The Use of Mathematical Models

How well do animal responses to environmental agents predict human responses? Sometimes, quite well; for example, almost all of the known human carcinogens are also carcinogenic in animals. On the other hand, risk assessment in animals has sometimes led us astray – saccharine was at one time banned for human use because it was found that this substance produces bladder cancers in rodents. We now know that this response is peculiar to the rat – many epidemiological studies have failed to find an **association** between bladder cancer and saccharine use in humans. Furthermore, we now understand the explanation for this species difference; rats excrete a protein into the urine that in the presence of saccharine produces bladder stones that, in turn, produce cancer. Humans do not excrete such a protein.

Another example is thalidomide, the sedative that is now known to produce shortened extremities in the fetuses of women given the drug during pregnancy. Studies in rats prior to marketing the drug failed to show such effects (rabbits do show effects similar to those in humans).

Why are very high doses used in animal experiments? Because the great majority of chemical carcinogens produce such weak effects that an effect can only be demonstrated by subjecting the animals to near-toxic levels. The practice of high dose testing in animals, and the interpretation of results from such experiments, is controversial; it is based on the assumption that the same mechanisms operate at high and at low doses. Bruce Ames, professor of biochemistry at the University of California, Berkeley, claims that chemicals administered at such high doses create cancers by a different process than that which would operate at usual doses, and therefore cancer rates observed at very high doses are not an appropriate means of carcinogen testing (Am90).

Mathematical modeling, used for extrapolation from high-dose animal data to human risks, is a matter of judgment and controversy. The model chosen can lead to vastly different estimates of risk at low levels of exposure, as shown in Figure 6.II, taken from the work of biostatistician Kenny Crump (Cr85). The figure shows five different models, all based on the same data for benzopyrene carcinogenesis as found in studies of mice. These different models vary greatly in their prediction of risk. In addition to the prediction of no risk at all (threshold model), the different models predict a numerical range of risks that differ by 100,000 fold. Clearly, the judgments of the analyst and the risk manager in choosing the appropriate model for regulatory purposes will have as much influence on the final risk estimate as the experimental data itself. Individuals are likely to have very different decision rules on these matters.

Natural Carcinogens

A common misperception is that all cancer-causing agents are of industrial origin, whereas chemicals of natural origin, such as those in food, are harmless. As Bruce Ames has repeatedly written, the vast bulk of chemicals ingested by humans are of natural origin. That is, they are synthesized by living things (plants and animals). When tested in the laboratory, many of these natural chemicals are carcinogenic. Many plants synthesize chemical pesticides as a means of protection against insect predators that prey upon them. As a consequence, more than 99.99% of the pesticides that we consume are of

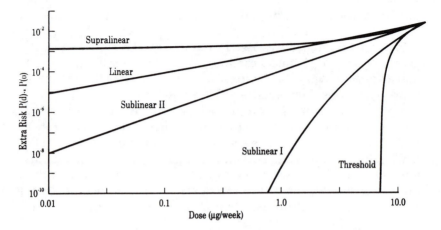

Figure 6.II   Results of Alternative Extrapolation Models for the Same Data From a Benzopyrene Carcinogenesis Experiment With Mice

natural origin. Half of these natural pesticides have been shown to be carcinogenic when tested in rats (Am90).

To illustrate the fact that carcinogens of natural origin are common in the diet, the American Council on Science and Health has published a Thanksgiving holiday menu, listing the carcinogenic or toxic ingredients in each of the foodstuffs. These are shown in Table 6.1.

Table 6.1   Holiday Menu—With Toxic or Carcinogenic Ingredients

Serving	Toxic or Carcinogenic Ingedients
Cream of mushroom soup	Hydrazines
Carrots	Carototoxin, myristicin, isoflavones, nitrate
Radishes	Glucosonoloates, nitrate
Cherry tomatoes	Hydrogen peroxide, querccetin glycocides, tomatine
Celery	Nitrate, psoralens
Assorted nuts	Aflatoxins
Roast turkey	Heterocyclic amines, malonaldehyde
Bread stuffing	Benzopyrene, di and tri sulfides, ethly carbamate, furan derivatives, dihydrazines, psoralens, safrole
Cranberry sauce	Eugenol, furan derivatives
Lima beans	**Cyanogenic glycosides**
Broccoli	Alkyl isothyocyanate
Baked potato	Amylase inhibitors, arsenic, chaconine, isoflavones, solanine
Pumpkin pie	Myristicine, nitrate, safrole
Apple pie	Acetaldehyde isoflavones, quercetin, safrole
Coffee	Benzopyrene, caffeine, chlorogenic acid, methylglyoxyl, tannins
Red wine	Alcohol, ethyl carbamate, methylglyoxal, tannins, tyramine

The point that this illustration makes is not that turkey dinners cause cancer, but rather that the methods we use to identify carcinogens, exposing animals at very high doses over a lifetime, are very likely to show positive results. If those same methods are applied to natural ingredients in the diet, then many common dietary ingredients are suspect carcinogens.

Summing the Risks and Benefits

An important but often overlooked point in risk assessment is that while exposure to a certain agent may increase the risk of a particular disease, other health risks may simultaneously be reduced by that very same exposure. The point was powerfully made in a study conducted by Graham Golditz and Anna Tosteson of Brigham and Women's Hospital in Boston. They found that while estrogen-replacement therapy might increase a woman's chance of developing breast cancer, that risk was more than balanced by the protection conferred by the drug against heart disease and osteoporosis; both of these conditions were decreased among those taking estrogens. In quantitative terms, those taking estrogens experienced an average life shortening of 15 days, but the life lengthening resulting from the reduction in other disease conditions produced a net benefit equivalent to an overall 27-day increase in life expectancy (NYT93). This kind of balancing of benefits and risks is faced by physicians daily, since almost all medical procedures carry some risks as well as benefits.The balancing of benefits and risks could become important in the management of EMF. For example, bringing transmission lines closer together could reduce magnetic fields, but create increased risks for linemen; altering grounding systems in homes could reduce magnetic fields, but increase the risk of electric shock to inhabitants of the house.

Risk Management

Once a risk has been established and quantified, the first part of the risk assessment process is completed; now the question becomes— what do we as a society do about it—how do we manage the risk?

Those who manage risk, either for the public, i.e., regulators or public health officials, or for ourselves (each of us is our own personal risk manager) ask questions such as: What is the magnitude of a risk? What would be the costs of avoiding the risks? What risks are associated with alternatives to the use of that agent or process?

Sometimes the answer will be that we do nothing at all, because the risk is too small, too uncertain, or too expensive to reduce, or because the benefits are too great (the use of the automobile may be an example). Sometimes the answer will be to remove that risk altogether. What other options exist? How are such decisions made?

Cost-Benefit Analysis

While comparisons of risks are sometimes useful in risk management, it is also sometimes useful to compare the risks of a technology or the use of an agent (such as pesticides) with the benefits associated with the use of that agent or technology. Cost-benefit analysis is a technique used to examine those costs and benefits in a systematic fashion. Take, for example, the desirability of a large engineering project such as a hydroelectric dam. Clearly, a good deal of agricultural potential, aesthetic value, and other benefits of existing land are destroyed by the construction of the dam. The designer of the project calculates, usually in dollars, the benefits of the dam, including flood control, recreation and commercial use, and compares those benefits with the costs incurred, including the acquisition of the land and the costs of construction. If the equation shows a net benefit, the project achieves some justification.

Ideally, such a calculus provides an objective measure of costs and benefits. In reality, judgments are necessarily subjective and often contentious. Each of the stakeholders (the impacted parties) may well have different views of both the benefits and the costs.

Cost-benefit analysis has been adopted for environmental control as well as for engineering projects. Here the question becomes, "How much benefit, in terms of health or premature deaths avoided, or aesthetic value, do we obtain by the expense of reducing pollution?" Just as with engineering projects, judgments are likely to differ here as well. One difficulty with the use a cost-benefit approach to environmental control is that it is often extremely difficult to assess the dollar values (or any other common metric) of both the costs and benefits and to convert them into equivalent units. Owners of the property or technology are likely to disagree about both the costs and the benefits to be achieved by a proposed management strategy.

There is another problem with cost-benefit analysis: the risks may not be experienced by the same population that receives the benefits. For example, a hydroelectric project may show aggregate benefits that far outweigh the aggregate risks, but the benefits, in terms of cheaper electric rates, may go to people in a distant city while the greatest risks are borne by those who live below the dam. But then, other people live near the airport used by the persons living near the dam, and so forth. We have no satisfactory means of fairly allocating each of these risks.

The Value of Life

Questions about risk management frequently lead to a very sensitive question: what is the value of a life? How much are we willing to spend to avoid a premature death? In our society, many people are repelled by the notion of putting a price on human life. Since we like to think that life is priceless, putting a price on it suggests a certain callousness, a commercialization of life. Yet, implicitly or explicitly, we do put a price on the value of life each time we consider safety measures. For example, let us consider a particularly dangerous rail-road crossing where one death per year, on average, occurs. The cost of building an underpass is $5 million. Over 50 years, 50 accidental deaths would be avoided at a cost of $100,000 per life saved (ignoring discounting). Is that worth it, or not? Obviously, the issue is likely to be considerably more complicated. An underpass may have benefits other than safety—convenience, for example—and other costs, such as injuries involved in construction of the underpass.

Calculation of the cost-effectiveness of health and safety programs can also be useful to government in comparing the value of these programs with other societal needs. After all, these costs do compete with other human needs such as education, housing, or environmental needs. When, as noted by Philip Abelson, former editor of *Science* magazine, we are spending an estimated $15 billion per life saved in the Superfund program, we know that other societal needs are being short-changed (Ab92). With respect to EMF, research must determine whether there is a risk from exposure, and if a risk does exist, how large it is, how many people are likely to be affected, and the most cost-effective means of reducing that risk.

Summary

In attempting to systematically identify and quantify risks, a system of risk assessment has been developed. When applied to risks to health, this methodology involves certain steps – hazard identification, dose-response assessment, exposure assessment, and risk characterization. Although public perception is always likely to influence regulatory decision-making, the process of risk assessment is intended to provide objective information necessary to risk management, a process of balancing risks and benefits.

When the risks are uncertain, and the benefits great, as with electricity and EMF, then risk assessment and management are doubly difficult. We shall return to this issue in the final chapter.

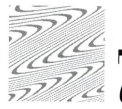

7

Epidemiology– a History

A possible linkage between EMF and human cancer is based mostly on epidemiological evidence. For that reason, and because epidemiology is so central to risk assessment generally, this chapter and the next provide an introduction to the subject. In this chapter, some of the highlights of epidemiological history are examined. In the next chapter are outlined some of the techniques of epidemiological studies—how they are done, together with some guidelines for interpreting epidemiological studies.

Epidemiology—A Definition

Some diseases appear to occur almost randomly among members of the population, without regard for the young or the old, the weak or the strong. The influenza epidemic of 1918–1920 is an example; the disease and death occurred among young healthy soldiers equally with others, both younger and older. The common cold is another example.

With most diseases, however, certain segments of the population seem to be unusually vulnerable. Measles is most common among

children, lung cancer is much more common among cigarette smokers, and, at least in the United States, AIDS occurs predominantly
among homosexuals or intravenous drug users.

Epidemiology is the science that attempts to understand the
causes of disease through recognition of these patterns.

What Does "Causation" Mean?

Some scientists object to the use of the word "cause" in epidemiological research, reserving the word for cases where a certain condition *always* leads to a particular outcome. For example, an increase in temperature always leads to an expansion
of the mercury in the thermometer—the outcome is highly
predictable and the temperature rise can rightly be said to
cause the expansion of the mercury. On the other hand, while
cigarette smoking sometimes leads to lung cancer, it does not
always do so; therefore (in this view), cigarette smoking is
better referred to as a **"risk factor"** for lung cancer, rather
than a cause of lung cancer.

Scientific methods can be very accurate in predicting the
behavior of simple systems, such as mercury thermometers.
Scientific methods are much less useful when attempting to
understand and predict the behavior of complex systems,
such as that of the weather, or of the human body. People have
sometimes said, "If we can send a man to the moon, we can
prevent cancer." But there are enormous differences in com-
plexity between sending a rocket aloft and understanding the
reaction of individual human beings to a complex mixture
such as tobacco smoke. While we may improve our understanding of the latter process, it is likely that we will never understand the process well enough to predict human responses to drugs or environmental agents with the same degree of accuracy that we can predict the response of the mercury thermometer to temperature change.

Some Early Epidemiological Discoveries

Historically, medical opinion on the causes of disease was based on
the writing of authority figures such as Galen, a Greek physician of
the second century, AD. For well over 1000 years, whatever Galen

had written about the origins of disease was unquestioned—medical thinking was frozen in time. Only in the last few hundred years have we begun to question medical authority, to interest ourselves in statistics, i.e., to observe how many people there are, how many are being born, how many are dying, how many persons are in each age group—and in drawing conclusions about the causes of disease on the basis of who is sick and who is not.

Why was there so little interest in exploring the causes of disease? It was because until recently it was believed that everything was a matter of "fate," or "the will of God." That earthly events such as epidemics are the result of physical or biological laws that people can understand and prevent is a relatively new departure in human thinking.

James Lind and Scurvy

Many of the early epidemiological discoveries arose from astute observations, often no more than the hunches of shrewd physicians who saw relationships in the behavior or lifestyle of patients with certain diseases. For example, James Lind, a British physician (1716–1794), noted that following long sea voyages, sailors were likely to develop the cluster of symptoms now known as scurvy. Lind speculated that this was the result of the monotonous and limited diet provided sailors on long sea voyages. To test his hypothesis, he studied 12 sailors on board his ship bound for Plymouth, England, all sick with scurvy. He divided them into six different treatment groups of two each, one of which was fed with sea water, one with vinegar, one with "cyder," one with elixir vitriol, one with a mixture of herbs, and the last with oranges and lemons. This was the result, in Lind's own words:

"The consequence was, that the most sudden and visible good effects were perceived from the use of the oranges and lemons; one of those who had taken them being at the end of six days fit for duty. The spots were not at that time quite off his body, nor his gums sound, but without any other medicine, than a gargarism of elixir vitriol, he became quite healthy before we came into Plymouth, which was on the 16th June. The other was the best recovered of any in his condition; and being now deemed pretty well, was appointed nurse to the rest of the sick"(Li80).

John Snow and Cholera

Another example of a shrewd observation, this time related to the role of microorganisms in disease causation, was also that of a practicing physician— John Snow (1813–1858), a London physician and anesthetist (he delivered two of Queen Victoria's children using chloroform anesthesia). Snow made some brilliant deductions regarding the street addresses of cases of cholera during a mid-19th century epidemic in London. He noted that the disease occurred more commonly among clients of a certain water company, Southwark and Vauxhall, which drew its water supplies from the Thames River at a point where the river was heavily contaminated. There was a lower rate of disease among clients of the competing Lambeth water company, which drew its water from a less-contaminated portion of the river. He conducted a study, summarized in table 7.I.

There was other information pointing to drinking water as the cause of the cholera; in Snow's words:

"There is a brewery in Broad Street, near to the pump and on perceiving that no brewer's men were registered as having died of cholera, I called on Mr. Huggins, the proprietor. He informed me that there were about seventy workmen employed in the brewery, and that none of them had suffered from cholera, at least in the severe form, only two having been indisposed, and that not seriously, at the time the disease prevailed. The men were allowed a certain amount of malt liquor, and Mr. Huggins believes they do not drink water at all; and he is quite certain that the workmen never obtained water from the pump in the street. There is a deep well in the brewery, in addition to the New River water." (Sn49)

Although these observations were made before the discovery of bacteria as a cause of disease, Snow concluded that it was the water that was responsible for the disease. He proved his case when he padlocked an offending well, the Broad Street pump (now an obliga-

Table 7.1 Death Rates From Cholera, by Source of Drinking Water

Water Supply Company	Deaths per 10,000 Houses
Southwark and Vauxhall	315
Lambeth Company	37
Rest of London	59

tory stop for epidemiologists visiting London), thereby ending the epidemic.

Note that in both of these observations a statistical association was not sufficient to prove the case; only through experiment (feeding oranges and lemons, capping the well) was causation proven.

These observations, Lind's insight regarding the role of fresh fruits and vegetables in scurvy and Snow's discovery of the role of contaminated water in cholera, were both but steps in the understanding of causation in these diseases. Only later was it further understood that ascorbic acid (vitamin C) is deficient in people with scurvy and that the cholera vibrio is the specific cause of the disease, cholera. We shall understand still more in the future about other contributing causes of these diseases.

Occupational Epidemiology

Much of the early epidemiological work hardly required great scientific insights—the association between occupation and disease was often blatantly obvious. When the majority of persons engaged in the making of hats became psychotic (mercury intoxication), when the majority of stone grinders died at a very young age of lung disease (silicosis), and when the bones of young girls who had been radium dial painters began crumbling (radium intoxication), the causes were tragically obvious. It was only the identification of the specific toxic agent responsible for these dreadful illnesses that required scientific detective work.

All of these examples illustrate the importance of disease clusters in expanding knowledge of the environmental sources of human disease. Cluster is defined as an unusual occurrence of disease in a particular segment of the population. The interpretation of apparent clusters, particularly neighborhood clusters, is tricky (Are they real or only chance associations?), as we shall see in Chapter 11.

Cancer Epidemiology

One of the first observations of cancer in an occupational population was that made by Percival Pott, a British physician who practiced surgery in London in the eighteenth century. Pott observed an unusually frequent incidence of cancer of the scrotum in young boys employed to clean chimneys. Because the children inevitably became covered with coal dust, and because particles of the dust would remain for long periods in contact with skin between the folds of the scrotum, cancers of the scrotum were common. This was perhaps the first observation of the carcinogenicity of coal tars, a phenomenon not unrelated to the carcinogenicity of tobacco tars in the lungs of cigarette smokers. The tragedy was that regular bathing, had it been available to these children, could have prevented the cancers.

A last historical example is the work of Arthur Herbst, a Massachusetts gynecologist who became interested in the relatively rare cancer of the vagina when he became aware of eight young women with the disease treated in the Boston area within a relatively short period of time (He88). These eight cases, observed by a single physician, were more than had been reported previously throughout recorded medical history. Herbst noted that the mothers of these women had a history of having been treated with the drug diethylstilbestrol (DES) during pregnancy. DES was at one time given to very large numbers of women who had experienced recurrent miscarriages. The drug is a close relative of the hormone estrogen, and was thought to be useful in permitting the pregnancy to go to completion. Since the discontinuation of DES treatment of pregnant women, vaginal cancer has dramatically declined in incidence

Interestingly, although the risk of vaginal cancer is very much increased among the daughters of women treated with DES (by several hundred fold), vaginal cancer occurs in only one in a thousand women exposed to DES during fetal life. In other words, even though the risk relative to untreated women is very great, the absolute risk is still very small—multiplying a very small risk by several hundred fold is still a very small risk. While the exposure to the drug is an almost necessary precondition, it is generally not sufficient to produce the disease. Clearly, other factors, possibly including genetic predisposition, mother's health status, and exposure to other chemicals, are necessary.

Environmental Epidemiology

Just as bacterial contamination of the environment can cause disease, so too can physical and chemical agents in the environment (air, water, or food). The most persuasive evidence of this comes from studies, such as those cited above, linking high and prolonged exposures in the workplace to human diseases.

Outside of the workplace, exposures are less frequent and of lower concentration, and clear-cut examples of environmentally induced disease are fewer. Deaths from respiratory and heart disease related to air pollution from the combustion of fossil fuels are one example. One of the best-documented episodes occurred in London in 1962, where approximately 4000 deaths occurred during a particularly intense five-day period of air pollution. The epidemic was not recognized until after the event, when, as remembered by Robert Waller, a researcher at London's St. Bartholomew's Hospital, "undertakers began running out of coffins and florists out of flowers." (Wa92b)

Not all alleged clusters of disease attributed to pollution are as clear-cut as the London smog example. One of the most widely publicized was that at Love Canal, New York. Fears of serious health effects were based on a single epidemiological study (the Paigen study) which created sufficient anxiety that 2500 residents were evacuated. Later, a scientific review was conducted by a panel headed by Lewis Thomas, chancellor of the Sloan-Kettering Cancer Center, which stated that the study:

> ". . . falls far short of the mark as an exercise in epidemiology...(and) her data cannot be taken as scientific evidence for her conclusions. The study is based on largely anecdotal information provided by questionnaires submitted to a narrowly selected group of residents. There are inadequate control groups, the illnesses cited as caused by chemical pollution were not medically validated...The panel finds the Paigen report literally impossible to interpret. It cannot be taken seriously as a piece of sound epidemiological research, but it does have the impact of polemic (Fu93)."

One strategy for examining the possible effects of industrial chemicals on cancer rates has been the examination of cancer mortality rates over recent decades. While the production of industrial chemicals has risen enormously, incidence rates for many cancer types have increased (Ca94). This has been interpreted by some to signal the effect of chemical carcinogens in the environment.

Changes in age-specific cancer mortality rates over the 25 years from 1950 to 1985 are shown in Table 7.2, both for all cancers and for all cancers minus lung cancer. (Cancer rates minus those for lung cancer are shown separately since the later are largely attributable to cigarette smoking). Note that the greatest declines are for the youn-

Table 7.2   Thirty Five Year Trends in Cancer Mortality

	Cancer Mortality Rates per 100,000 Persons All races, both sexes					
	All Sites			All Sites Minus Lung		
	1950	1985	Percent Change	1950	1985	Percent Change
0– 4	11.0	3.6	-67.3	10.9	3.6	-67.0
5–14	6.6	3.5	-47.0	6.5	3.5	-46.2
15–24	8.5	5.3	-37.6	8.3	5.3	-36.1
25–34	19.6	12.8	-34.7	18.9	12.2	-35.4
35–44	63.9	48.2	-24.6	59.3	39.8	-32.9
45–54	174.7	169.3	-3.1	154.4	118.9	-23.0
55–64	392.0	441.3	12.6	343.1	292.2	-14.8
65–74	695.0	848.0	22.0	636.1	586.0	-7.9
75–84	1147.5	1290.2	12.4	1092.4	1004.2	-8.1
85+	1444.8	1596.2	10.5	1401.9	1403.5	0.1
All ages	157.0	171.3	9.1	144.0	124.8	-13.3

gest age groups. The elderly have not experienced a similar decline (So89).

There are two explanations for the observations of rising incidence rates at a time when mortality rates are steady or declining. The first is that mortality rates have remained stable, in spite of rising incidence rates, because of improved therapy. The other possible explanation (the two are not mutually exclusive) is that rising incidence rates are only a reflection of improved medical surveillance—more persons being seen by physicians who have improved technological means for detecting cancer.

The most comprehensive study of the causes of human cancer was conducted by Sir Richard Doll and Richard Peto. They estimate that only a very small percentage of cancer can arise from chemical or physical pollution of the environement (Do81). Others in the scientific community are in agreement. Writing in _Science_ magazine, cancer epidemiologists Brian Henderson, Ronald Ross, and Malcolm Pike assert that, "The widespread public perception that environmental pollution is a major cancer hazard is incorrect" (He81). A report of the Council on Scientific Affairs of the American Medical Association concludes: "one of the most comprehensive reviews of the epidemiologic literature ever conducted concluded that synthetic chemicals are not a significant cause of human cancer, except in isolated instances of occupational exposure." (AMA93).

Summary

Epidemiology has been and continues to be a powerful tool for the discovery of the causes of disease when risks are relatively large, when the disease of concern is specific and easily identified (e.g., scurvy, vaginal cancer, lung cancer), and when adequate tools for exposure assessment are available.

In the next chapter, we shall look more closely at the methodology of epidemiology and ask how one can make judgments about causation, in contrast with statistical association.

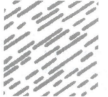

8

Epidemiology– a Guide to Establishing Cause

Most humans have difficulty with uncertainty—we need explanations. Why do crops fail? Why was the baby born deformed? Why did the barn burn down? Why are we here? From where did we come? What is "The Truth?"

The need to understand the truth is so great that if explanations do not exist, we invent them. As Isaac Asimov put it: "Inspect every piece of pseudoscience, and you will find a security blanket, a thumb to suck, a skirt to hold. What have we to offer in exchange? Uncertainty! Insecurity!" (As92)

Different cultures go about searching for the truth in different ways. Many depend on introspection, or on studying scriptures. In modern times, we also depend on what we call the scientific method, on observation and experiment.

Much truth is not eternal but ephemeral. All wise men once said that the sun rotates around the earth. We now know the reverse to be true. Until recently, geologists believed that the continents had always existed where they are now found. Now we believe in plate tectonics—that the continents have drifted over the surface of the globe—and are still drifting. In the medical world, that which is gospel today is gone tomorrow. Tonsillectomies were routinely prescribed for the majority of children until thirty or forty years ago when it became clear how often useless and even dangerous this procedure could be. Most children who have experienced a tonsillectomy never forget the awful terror.

As ephemeral as truth may be, within the scientific method, there is general agreement on tests of truth. This chapter describes the tests applied to epidemiological studies to understand the causes of human disease.

Disease Causation

Robert Koch (1843–1910), a German pathologist and winner of the Nobel Prize (1905), took a great interest in the matter of the role of microorganisms in the causation of infectious disease, and formulated certain criteria for assigning a causal role in a specific disease to a particular organism. i.e., the tubercle bacillus as the causal agent of tuberculosis. His criteria were:

- The suspect organism must be found in *all* patients with the disease.

- The organism must not be found in patients *without* the disease.

- Under experimental conditions in the laboratory, injections of the organism into animals must be able to produce the disease.

- Transmitting the organism from an infected animal to another animal must be associated with the production of the disease in the second animal, i.e., it must be transmissible.

We now know that these criteria are far too stringent. The central thesis of what became known as Koch's postulates is that one organism produces only one disease, and *always* produces that disease. Neither of these conclusions need be true. Polio and tuberculosis are examples: in both cases, many people will be *infected*, but only a few will develop *disease*. Many healthy persons can be found who have streptococcus in their throats without the disease, strep throat.

Furthermore, a single organism may cause different diseases in different populations. The Epstein-Barr virus is an example, producing cancer (Burkitt's lymphoma) in African children, but the relatively benign infectious mononucleosis among young Americans.

Chronic disease epidemiology is considerably more difficult than is the epidemiologic study of the acute infectious diseases, since the chronic diseases often appear to have multiple, rather than a single, causal agent.

Given these difficulties and complexities, how does the epidemiologist arrive at conclusions regarding disease causation?

Epidemiology in a Few Easy Lessons

There are a number of methods for conducting an epidemiological study. Let us consider briefly three that are most commonly used: the **ecological** study (not to be confused with the more common use of the word), the **case-control** study, and the **cohort** study.

The Ecological Study.   An ecological study is one in which groups, rather than individuals, are compared. One often sees such correlations in international studies. For example, there is a strong correlation of beer consumption with rectal cancer in different countries (Czechoslovakia has the highest rate of both).

The problem with ecological studies is that we do not know whether the individuals with disease are representative of the population as a whole. In the example above, are the individuals with rectal cancers heavy beer drinkers? To put it another way, an ecological study does not provide us with information on exposure *in the individual*. Nevertheless, ecologic studies are cheap and easy to do. Often the can be done with easily available data. They have their greatest use in generating hypotheses, but are less valuable in proving causation.

As we shall see, ecological studies have been widely used in the study of cancer among electrical workers, i.e., those whose job titles suggest exposure to EMF (e.g., electricians, electronic assemblers).

The Case-Control Study.   This commonly used design has been frequently used in studying EMF and childhood cancer; the Wertheimer-Leeper and the Savitz studies mentioned in an earlier chapter are examples of case-control studies.

"Cases" are those subjects with the disease in question. "Controls" are those without the disease who are selected for the purpose of comparison. Basically, the logic here is to compare the *exposures* of the cases with that of the controls. Controls are usually matched with cases according to several variables which may include: age, gender, social class, or others. If the exposure of the cases is significantly greater than that of the controls, then the investigator may conclude that the exposure may have *caused* the disease in the cases.

While the case-control study has certain advantages over the ecological study, problems remain. One of these is exposure assessment. Frequently, as with EMF, the epidemiologist is in a position of having to reconstruct past exposures from scanty evidence. Another problem is the selection of controls; if the controls are not chosen from the same community or cohort as the cases, then serious errors can arise in the interpretation of such comparisons.

The Cohort Study.   A cohort is any group of persons that has some common attribute. For example, all employees of a particular company, all persons born in the same year, or all persons living in the same community might constitute a cohort. A cohort study, the study of exposure and health oucomes in a single population or cohort, may be retrospective, i.e., examine the past experience of a cohort, or may be prospective. In the latter case, the cohort is first identified and then observed over some subsequent period of time.

Retrospective cohort studies.   Cohort studies are frequently designed to assess risk among employees of a single industry or company who have been exposed for some years to a particular industrial environment. These investigations suffer form the same problem of the case-control study, namely, the retrospective assessment of exposure.

The many studies of lung cancer among uranium miners are examples of retrospective cohort studies. In the uranium miner studies, measurements of air concentrations of radon gas are made, the duration of employment of the miner in that mine is then used to assign a lifetime exposure to that miner. However, the environment within that mine may have changed considerably over the years, due to new mining techniques and changes in ventilation. Or, the mine where the miner worked may no longer be actively mined. Under these conditions, estimates of exposure may be highly unreliable.

Nevertheless, a retrospective cohort study is generally considered to provide more valid information regarding causation than a case-control study, since it is less likely to be **biased**, particularly in the selection of controls, since there are no controls – the comparison of disease in the cases is with all other members of the cohort (e.g., other uranium miners).

The Prospective Cohort Study.   These studies are generally considered to be the gold standard for inferring causality. The design is superior because it provides the potential for the best exposure assessment (prior to the development of disease) and the best assessment of disease outcome.

The distinct advantage of the case-control study is the ease with which cases can be assembled. In contrast, with rare diseases such as the childhood leukemias, a cohort study , in order to generate sufficient numbers of cases to be significant, may require the identification of a very large cohort for study and exposure assessment. It can be done, but often at very large cost.

Two examples of prospective cohort studies are the studies of the survivors of the atomic bombings of Japan and the Framingham study of heart disease among the citizens of a small Massachusetts town. In the former case, the health of some 100,000 survivors has now been studied for almost 50 years, the health of those heavily exposed compared with those with lesser exposures to radiation. In the Framingham study, a great number of risk factors for heart disease (e.g., smoking, diet, exercise) have been studied in this same population over several decades.

These, then, are the major types of epidemiological study. Now we turn to consideration of some other issues in evaluating epidemiological studies: bias and confounding, both of which can lead to distorting the results of a study.

Distinguishing Chance Association From Causal Associations

A common mistake is to confuse things that coexist in time or space through chance alone from those that occur together because one causes the other. Correlations are commonly found in comparing two populations. It is a very natural thing to confuse correlation with causation: if two things occur together, then we easily fall into the trap of assuming that one must be *causing* the other. Distinguishing the two phenomena, association and causation, is not always easy. Sometimes it is not clear whether A is causing B, B is causing A, something else is causing A and B, or finally, A and B are not causally related at all.

Let us look at an illustrative example. A decline in the numbers of storks nesting in Scandinavia has been noted during the past few decades. A decline has also been noted in the Scandinavian birth rate.

What is the relationship? According to the theory that storks bring babies, the decline in the stork population is the cause of the decline in
births (A causes B). Another possible explanation is that babies attract
storks (B causes A). Perhaps the sight of white diapers hanging on
clothes lines is attractive to storks; the fewer the diapers, the fewer the
storks. A more likely explanation is that the two phenomena, the declines in storks and babies, are the result of some third factor, possibly
the rise of modern civilization, with its smaller families and its en-
croachment on stork nesting sites (C causes A and B). The last possibility is that the decline in the stork and the baby populations have nothing
at all to do with each other (A unrelated to B). How can one be sure?

An example of an association the meaning of which is mysterious
was discovered by sports writer Leonard Koppett. He has noted that
the winning team of the Super Bowl is highly predictive of stock market performance for the year. Koppett asserts that if the Super Bowl is
won by a team that was formerly a member of the American Football
League, the stock market will show a loss for the year; whereas if the
winning team was a member of the National Football League prior to
the merger of the two leagues, the market will go up that year. This
has proven to be true in 26 of the past 27 years. "The beauty of the situation," Koppett said, "is that one cannot even imagine any conceiv-
able explanation for it, except randomness" (Ko93).

Another example of the kinds of unexplainable correlations that
occasionally turn up is the work of two Michigan researchers, Bar-
nett Rosenberg and David Juckett. These men undertook an examination of the life spans of U.S. Congressmen, born prior to 1900.
They chose Congressmen because there are good records of birth
and death dates. What they found was a gentle oscillation in the
number of years of life, rising over several years, and then falling
over a few years. Puzzled by this, they examined the correlation between sunspot activity and longevity of the legislators, and found a
high degree of correlation, but only when they used—not the date of
birth—but the date of birth minus twenty years. They interpret this
as showing an effect of sunspots on the health of the mother twenty
years prior to her pregnancy (Re93). Another explanation: the
association is totally without meaning and is an example of those
correlations that turn up when computers are available and when
one examines enough data.

Some Pitfalls in Epidemiology

In this next section, we first examine two common problems of epidemiological studies, **bias** and **confounding**, following which we shall look at measures of the strength of an association (in our case, the measure of risk), and then the issue of judging whether the association is statistically significant.

Bias

As a term used by epidemiologists, bias has a somewhat different meaning than it does in everyday usage, where bias has a meaning akin to prejudice. In epidemiological studies, any errors in evaluating the relationship between exposure and health outcomes are known as sources of bias, which can either mask or exaggerate an association.

For example, bias can occur in the selection of the study subjects, in the ways in which information is obtained, or in the ways in which disease is ascertained. It is widely recognized that patients with disease are more likely to remember exposure to agents thought to be responsible for that disease than are subjects who are in good health—an example of "recall bias."

A classical example of bias occurs in the study of heart disease among hospitalized subjects who might differ in many ways from the larger population of persons with that disease. Many patients who suffer heart attacks do not reach a hospital, either because they die before they reach the hospital, because the heart attack is not recognized, or because they are treated at home. Therefore, conclusions regarding heart disease based solely on the study of hospitalized patients could lead to imprecise conclusions regarding heart disease in general.

Another form of bias, associated not with the conduct of studies themselves, but rather with the publication of studies, is the so-called "**publication bias**." This results when only some studies are published and not all studies. This could occur if the investigators do not think a study worthy of publication, or if the editors of journals only accept studies with a certain result. For example, both investigators and journal editors are more likely to publish studies that find a positive result (i.e., where exposure is associated with an effect), than with negative studies. Since risk assessors reach conclusions on the basis of the balance of published studies, this bias could result in the false attribution of health effects when in fact none actually exists. Several studies of this phenomenon do indeed show that publication bias exists (Ea91).

The extent to which publication bias might involve EMF health studies is not known, but that it does occur to some degree seems likely. One reviewer notes that in conjunction with a study of leukemia among Canadian workers, reports of an increased risk among members of two electrical occupations, power and telephone linemen, was published (7 deaths compared with 2.9 expected), but reports of a decrease in risk among all other electrical workers were not published (9 deaths compared with 15.7 expected) (NRPB92 p94).

Confounding

Confounding refers to the possibility that what appears to be an association between disease and some suspect agent may be the result of unrecognized factors related to both the exposure and the health outcome (This is equivalent in my earlier example of A and B both being the result of some third unrecognized factor – industrialization causes both the decline in storks and the decline in births). An example: early studies of alcohol consumption and lung cancer show a strong association. Does alcohol cause the lung cancer, or was another factor confounding the association? Later studies showed that cigarette smoking is strongly associated with alcohol consumption. In fact, it is the cigarettes that are responsible for causing the lung cancer, not the alcohol.

Unfortunately, we know so little about the causes of childhood cancer that we can hardly even speculate, much less investigate, what factors might be confounding the relationship between wire codes and childhood cancer (see chapter 9). Several factors in addition to wire codes have been found associated with childhood cancer; these include traffic density (Sa89), infant feeding by bottle rather than breast (Da88), indoor use of pesticides (Lo91, Le95), consumption of hot dogs ((Sa94, Pe94b), and parental occupation in certain chemical or electrical industries (see Chapter 10). The evidence for any of these as a true causal factor for childhood cancer is weak. Moreover, most of these factors are not related to wire codes and therefore cannot explain the association of wire codes with childhood cancer.

There are techniques for avoiding confounding, especially when the possible influence of a third factor (such as cigarette smoking) is recognized. But if there is no knowledge of the possible operation of a third factor, then it may be impossible to adjust for this possible confounder. As we shall see, there may be some factor confounding the relationship between power lines and childhood cancer, but we know so little of the causes of childhood cancer that it is difficult to adjust for these possible confounders.

Measures of Risk

Unfortunately, there is no single means of characterizing the magnitude of the risk of disease. Rather, there are a variety of measures, each of which has some usefulness. Characterizing risk is something like the old parable about several blind men, using their hands alone, trying to understand the shape of an elephant. One man feels the trunk, another feels the tail, and a third feels a leg. Each of them comes away with a very different impression of an elephant, yet they are all correct. Each of them has seen one valid but incomplete attribute of an elephant.

Epidemiological studies not only produce evidence of an increase (or decrease) in risk, but also provide some measure of the magnitude of that risk as well. Very commonly, a **risk ratio** , that is, the risk of disease in an exposed population, compared with the risk of that disease in an unexposed population, is used to assess the magnitude of risk. If the source of the risk ratio is a cohort study, the statistic produced is known as a **relative risk,** whereas the case-control study produces a statistic known as an **odds ratio**.

Relative Risk. If, for example, the rate of lung cancer deaths among cigarette smokers were found to be 190 per 100,000 persons, and the death rate among nonsmokers were found to be 19 per 100,000, the relative mortality risk would be: 190/19=10, indicating that the risk of lung cancer death among smokers is 10 times higher than among nonsmokers. A relative risk of 1.0 would be interpreted as showing no increase in risk among the exposed.

It should always be remembered that the risk ratio is a ratio, and does not tell us much about the absolute risk. That is, if the natural risk is very small, then even an experience or exposure that produces a doubling of risk still produces an absolute risk that remains very small. For example, suppose that the risk of being struck by lightning is one in a million per year. Suppose that living in a certain location where electrical storms doubles the risk (a risk ratio of 2.0). The risk of one in 500,000 per year is still small enough that most of us would be willing to ignore the occurrence of electrical storms in choosing a place to live.

Odds Ratio.   Unlike a cohort study, which permits disease rates to be calculated, a case-control study, which compares *exposure rates* of cases and controls, does not permit the calculation of disease rates. It does permit the comparison of the odds of exposure among the cases with that of the controls.

The calculation of the odds ratio is as follows:

	Exposed	Unexposed
Cases	a	c
Controls	b	d

$$\text{Then,} \qquad \text{Odds Ratio} = \frac{a/c}{b/d} = \frac{ad}{bc}$$

The odds ratio is a reasonable estimate of the relative risk, and is interpreted in the same way as the relative risk; an odds ratio of 2.0 is interpreted as representing a relative risk of 2.0.

Relative risks or odds ratios are frequently used to examine possible increases in risk in certain segments of the population, such as members of social classes, racial groups, or geographic or occupational groups. It should be remembered that the odds ratio for the entire population will be 1.0, whereas the odds ratios for individual subgroups will often be higher or lower than 1.0. For example, in examining cancer rates among various job categories, half of the jobs examined will have odds ratios greater than one, whereas the other half will have odds ratios less than one. Whether an elevated or a reduced odds ratio is significant or not requires statistical testing, a matter explored in a later section.

Attributable Risk.   Another parameter of risk is the *number or percentage* of persons dying of a disease whose death was contributed to by exposure to the agent of interest. For example, the American Cancer Society estimates that cigarette smoking is responsible for 87% (133,000) of the 153,000 cancer deaths that occurred among Americans in 1984 (Ca94). How do they know this? The answer comes from knowledge of:

- the risk ratio for lung cancer among cigarette smokers (22 for males, 12 for females) and

- the number of persons who smoke (approximately 40% for males, 30% of females)

One formula for calculating attributable risk in a population exposed to a risk factor is

$$\frac{p(r - 1)}{1 + p(r - 1)}$$

where p = proportion of the population exposed

r = relative risk of those who are exposed

Statistical Significance

If a person were to flip a coin 10 times, it would not be surprising if heads came up more than 5 times. A result of 6 or even 7 heads would not be unexpected. Statistically, exactly 5 heads show up only 24.6% of the time when 10 coins are flipped. But with small numbers like 10, things rarely come out exactly as predicted on the basis of chance alone.

The kind of variability that appears with coin flipping also occurs in studies of health and disease in human populations. Given the likelihood that differences in rates of disease will occur in comparing two populations, how can the epidemiologist be sure that the difference is meaningful, i.e., likely due to the agent or exposure under study? In the cigarette example above, is the tenfold greater death rate among cigarette smokers real or just the result of random variation? One test that the epidemiologist applies is a statistical one: is the difference in the rates of the two populations small enough to be expected on the basis of chance alone (as in flipping coins), or is the difference so large as to plausibly exclude the operation of chance? **Statistical significance** is a matter of the likelihood of an outcome, not an absolute guarantee of causation.

Statisticians often use the "95% confidence level," by which they mean a difference this great will only occur by chance alone once in 20 times (The calculation is a technical one; the interested reader might consult Ba92 for further information). There is nothing magical about 95%; it would be foolish to accept a result as significant if it is at the 95% level and insignificant at the 94% level. If statisticians want a greater sense of security about statistical significance, they sometimes choose a 99% significance level, which suggests that the result will occur by chance only once in a hundred times. Through-out the remainder of this book, the reader may assume that the 95 percent confidence level is used to establish statistical significance, even though not specified.

Confidence Limits

Another test of the meaningfulness of an association is the use of con-fidence limits. When pollsters report their estimates of a candidate's approval, they will often say something like this: "President Smith has an approval rating of sixty-three percent. This estimate is accu-rate with a three percent margin of error." What this means is that (with a 95% significance level) the "approve" response will be some-where between 60 and 66%, ninety five percent of the time that such a study were done. By convention, the statistician would report this result like this: 63 (60–66). The 63 is known as the *point estimate* and the 60–66 are the *95 percent confidence limits.* which are normally shown in parentheses following the point estimate.

Confidence limits will narrow as the size of the study group in-creases. When the study group is small, the uncertainty about any conclusion reached will be relatively large. For example, in the pres-idential poll mentioned in the last paragraph, a larger polling sample might have produced the result 63 (62–64), narrower confidence lim-its, and less uncertainty about the estimate of 63%.

A special note regarding risk ratios or odds ratios: if the confi-dence limits include 1.0, i.e., no effect, then the statistician will inter-pret the result as not statistically significant, even though the risk estimate is greater than 1. For example, a risk estimate of 1.5 (0.9–2.1) will not be considered significant since a risk of 1.0, i.e., no risk, has not been excluded. In contrast, another study, also with a point esti-mate of 1.5, but with narrower confidence limts (such as 1.3–1.7) would be considered significant.

Reaching Conclusions

If increased disease rates are found in an exposed population, that increase could be the result of:

- a causal association between the exposure and the disease,
- a bias in the conduct of the study,

- confounding factors, or

- random variation—chance.

Given the pitfalls in epidemiological studies, how can one be sure that causation is real, and that one is not inadvertently encountering meaningless associations? In a famous lecture delivered in 1965, Sir Austin Bradford Hill suggested a number of tests that may be helpful in evaluating causation (Hi65). Among them were:

Magnitude and Precision of Risk. If exposure to the suspect agent produces a very great increase in disease, then a causal relationship is more likely. If the magnitude of the risk detected is small, then one is normally more cautious in accepting the association as a causal one. A two-fold increae in risk is often considered the lowest level of risk that can be confidently established through epidemiologic techniques. For example, the risk of breast cancer first found among women who drink alcoholic beverages was found in three studies to be twofold increased. On the basis of later studies, with relative risks less than two, however, the effect remains in doubt (Fe88).

Replication. Because there are opportunities for error (i.e., bias) in epidemiological studies, confidence in an association grows with the number and consistency of studies. If, as with cigarette smoking and lung cancer, the same conclusion of risk is reached in several studies conducted by different investigators in different parts of the world, then one may be more certain that the association is causal.

Exposure-Response Relationship. Did the investigator examine differences in disease among persons with different levels of exposure, and did those more-heavily exposed exhibit higher levels of disease? If the answer is affirmative, such evidence of a relationship between the dose and the response strengthens the conclusion that the relationship is a causal one and not spurious.

While the existence of an exposure-response relationship provides important evidence of a causal relationship, it is by no means foolproof. Consider the following example: There is a strong exposure-response relationship between cigarette smoking and suicide, as shown in the following table (Sm92).

Table 8.1.   Relative Rates of Suicide According to Cigarettes Smoked

Cigarettes per Day	Age-Adjusted Suicide Rate
0	1.00
10	1.36
20	1.88
30	2.31
60+	3.44

It hardly seems plausible that cigarette smoking *causes* people to kill themselves, particularly in view of the fact that there is also a relationship between cigarette smoking and homicide; the heavier the smoking, the greater the risks of homicide. Could cigarette smoking also cause murder? Almost certainly there is some confounder operating here, possibly social class, which is associated with both smoking and suicide.

Consistency.   Do each of the studies of a particular agent show, at least roughly, the same disease outcome with the same magnitude of risk? If different studies of an exposure show different disease outcomes, and if some studies show an effect whereas others do not, the evidence of causation is weakened.

Adequacy of Exposure Assessment.   Was the exposure objectively or subjectively measured? If, for example, the study is of the effect of diet, or alcohol, or drugs, dependence on the subjects memory is likely to be less reliable than an objective measure of consumption.

Adequacy of *Outcome* Ascertainment.   Just as a study can be flawed by poor ascertainment of exposure, so too can a study be flawed by poor ascertainment of the disease being studied. For example, if we are examining a study of brain cancer, did the investigators make certain that their cases were all brain cancers and not other diseases that might masquerade as brain cancers, e.g., cerebrovascular disease, metastatic lesions from other organs, abscesses, blood clots?

Plausibility.   Is there any biological basis on which to accept the association as causal? For an extreme example, we find an association between the use of telephones and the risk of heart disease. Is there any plausible explanation? Not really. Stress? Well, then we should conduct a study of stress and heart disease rather than depend on a surrogate, the telephone.

Does Elimination of the Alleged Cause Reduce the Risk?   In the example of the London cholera epidemic cited in the last chapter, we noted that Snow proved his suspicion that water contamination was the cause of cholera when he eliminated the cause by padlocking the offending well. This was followed by the disappearance of the disease. Such a demonstration is powerful proof that the association is causal.

Another particularly interesting example is the experience with the use of DES and vaginal cancer. As noted in the previous chapter, the rising number of cases of this disease in the 1960s and 1970s had raised suspicion about the drug, but even more-convincing proof of a causal relationship occurred when the use of the drug in the treatment of pregnancy disorders was stopped, followed by a decline in the incidence of vaginal cancer.

Bradford Hill warned that a check list such as this cannot provide indisputable evidence of causation. "What they can do is to help us make up our minds on the fundamental question—is there any other way of explaining the set of facts before us; is there any other answer equally or more likely than cause and effect?"

A Note About Excluding Risks

The epidemiologist searches for persons with increased, or decreased, levels of exposure to test whether there is a correlation with disease. Do people with high cholesterol have more heart disease? Do people with very low levels of cholesterol have very low levels of heart disease? While such questions, and their answers, can be useful in answering whether risks exist, the use of such techniques cannot be used to *exclude* risks. That is, our available methods will never allow us to say that cholesterol does not produce heart disease or that EMF does not produce cancer.

Summary

Epidemiology is a scientific method for examining possible risks in human populations. Many of the definitions and concepts developed in this chapter will be applied in the following chapters. The most important are as follows:

- **Risk.** The most general descriptor of risk, describing the likelihood of an increase or decrease in risk for a certain selected population in comparison with some suitable comparison
population.. For example: compared with non-smokers, cigarette smokers have an increased risk of cancer and heart disease.
This does not tell us how large is the risk.

- **Risk Ratio.** The mathematical comparison of the magnitude
of the risk in the study population, in comparison with a suitable
(or control) population. For example, the risk ratio for lung cancer among cigarette smokers is 10.0—a ten fold increase in risk.
Odds ratios and *relative risks* are both examples of risk ratios., the
former arising from a case-control study, and the latter from a
cohort study.

- **Significant Risk.** The risk ratio alone does not tell us whether the risk ratio is likely (or not) to have arisen by chance alone.
In order to reduce the likelihood that the risk ratio has arisen by
chance alone, tests of statistical significance are applied. The
usual test is the 95 percent confidence level. If by this criterion
the statistical test of significance shows that a given risk ratio is
significant, then the interpretation is that a difference this large
(between the exposed population and the control population)
is unlikely to occur by chance alone more often than once in
twenty studies. A risk ratio might appear to be rather high, e.g.,
5.0, and be statistically insignificant; in contrast, a rather low
risk ratio, e.g., 1.5, can be statistically significant. Statistical significance arises from the size of the population studied and the
magnitude of the risk found—the larger the number of cases
studied, and the greater the risk factor —the greater the likelihood that a given risk ratio will be significant.

- **Confidence Limits.** The 95 percent confidence limits are normally shown in parentheses following the risk ratio; for example, it might be written that cigarette smokers have a risk ratio of
10.0 (8.0–12.00), which implies that the test of significance shows
that 95 times out of a hundred, a study based on this size population would generate a risk ratio between 8.0 and 12.0. If the
confidence limits are narrow and the lower limit exceeds 1.0,
then the risk can be interpreted as valid, assuming that the study
is otherwise free of bias.

V
EMF AND CANCER

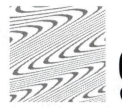

9

Residential Studies: EMF and Cancer

Two groups of epidemiological studies of cancer and EMF exposure exist—those of persons whose exposures arise from sources within and near the home, and those of persons exposed to EMF in the workplace. In this chapter the residential studies of EMF and cancer will be reviewed, and in the next chapter, the occupational studies will be discussed The residential studies have mostly, but not exclusively, examined childhood cancer.

It is not intended to exhaustively review and critique each of the many epidemiological studies of EMF and cancer that have been reported in the literature; rather, attention will be focused on those studies that have been the most important, either because of their size, the innovative nature of their methodology, or the significance of their findings. Comprehensive reviews of the literature can be found in many of the references found in Chapter 15.

Cancer in Children

Fortunately, in comparison with adults, children develop cancer rarely; there were an estimated 8,200 new cases in the United States in 1994, and an estimated 1,600 deaths (Ca94). Cancer occurs in about 1 child in 7000 per year, or in approximately 1 in 450 during the entire first 15 years of life. In contrast, almost 20% of adults reaching the age of 60 will have developed cancer during the previous 15 years (Gr85).

Cancer is not only much less common among children than among adults, it is also different in the organs and tissues involved. The most common childhood cancer is leukemia, followed by cancer of the brain and nervous system, the eye, the kidney, and the lymphatic system (Table 9.1).

What Causes Childhood Cancer?

Only a very few environmental agents are known with any certainty to increase the risk of childhood cancer. One is ionizing radiation, most extensively studied among the survivors of the atomic bombing of Hiroshima and Nagasaki.

Another is benzene, which causes leukemia in children as well as in adults. A cluster of cases of childhood leukemia was once seen in the Italian city of Vigevano, where it was the practice of workers in shoe manufacturing to bring home shoes to be treated with benzene-containing solvents. The vapors in the home were sufficient to produce leukemia in the children living in those homes.

Table 9.1   Childhood Cancer Incidence and Mortality Rates, 1985–89, per 100,000, United States (Ca 94)

Site	Incidence	Mortality
All sites	13.9	3.4
Acute lymphocytic leukemia	3.3	0.6
Bone and joint	0.7	0.1
Brain and nervous system	3.1	0.8
Hodgkin's disease	0.7	0.0
Kidney and renal pelvis	0.9	0.1
Non-Hodgkin's lymphoma	0.9	0.2
Soft tissue	0.8	0.2

Genetic factors are more evident in childhood cancer than in the adult disease (Kn88). The evidence comes from the frequent association of childhood cancer with known genetic defects. For example, children with Down's Syndrome (a complex of multiple birth defects, including mental retardation and short stature) have a rate of leukemia seven times that of other children. Children with hereditary immune deficiencies are particularly prone to cancer. In some cases, cancer risks are increased by one hundred fold. Children with xeroderma pigmentosa, a disease that very much increases sensitivity to sunlight, have a greatly increased risk of developing skin cancer.

It may be that environmental agents have little to do with most childhood cancer, although there has not been sufficient study of these diseases to be able to reach definitive conclusions on the matter.

The Leukemias

Leukemia is a disease of the blood-forming organs. It is marked by an overproduction of white blood cells, found in high concentration both in the bone marrow and in the circulating blood. These white cells are not normal cells—they are immature. Current thinking is that these malignant leukemia cells are unable to mature properly, and so accumulate in large numbers.

In normal persons, there are two predominant types of white cells, the myelocytes and the lymphocytes, which can be distinguished on the basis of their appearance under the microscope. The leukemias are often described by the predominant cell type involved in the disease; thus the two most common categories of leukemia are **myelogenous** and **lymphocytic**.

Leukemia is also characterized by the degree of malignancy, i.e., whether the leukemia is acute or chronic. The acute disease, the only type appearing in children, may be rapidly fatal if untreated, whereas the chronic disease, most commonly found in the elderly, may not be life-shortening, or even produce symptoms. The four most common forms of leukemia, then, are acute and chronic lymphocytic leukemia and acute and chronic myelogenous leukemia.

While leukemia is the commonest cancer among children, it is relatively uncommon among adults, accounting for an estimated 28,600 new cases in 1994, but that is only about 2.4% of all cancer (Ca94).

Some factors that have been shown to be risk factors for adult leukemia are exposures to benzene, ionizing radiation, cigarette smoking, paints, herbicides, and chemotherapeutic agents. There are also
certain occupations or industries that appear to be associated with
an increase in leukemia. They are farming, embalming, sawmill
work, and chemical manufacture (Sc82).

There is no known biological reason why leukemia should have a
stronger association with EMF exposure than with other cancer; nevertheless, there have been more studies of leukemia among persons with
occupational exposure to EMF than there have of any other cancer.

Childhood Residential Studies:

The approach followed here in describing the studies of EMF and
childhood cancer is historical—beginning with the first study (published in 1979) and then noting most of the subsequent studies in
chronological order.

The Wertheimer-Leeper Study

The first suggestion of an association of EMF with cancer arose from
the study of children conducted in Denver, Colorado, by Nancy
Wertheimer and Ed Leeper, published in 1979 (We79). Because there
was nothing in the literature that would otherwise support such an
association, the study met with considerable skepticism. Yet it raised
important questions, some of which remain unanswered today.

As Wertheimer tells the story, the Denver study was first con-
ceived when the matter of childhood cancer attracted her attention.
To educate herself, she drove to the neighborhoods and examined
the homes where the children with cancer had lived, looking for possible environmental clues. She noted what appeared to be an unusually high number of these homes in locations adjacent to pole-top
transformers, and particularly near power lines.

Intrigued by the possible association, Wertheimer sought the as-
sistance of the physicist, Leeper, with whom she developed a system
to estimate the magnetic fields inside homes—the "wire coding"
system described in Chapter 3.

The study began with an identification of all children who had
died from all types of cancer from 1950 to 1973. To be eligible for in-

clusion in the study, the child must have been born in Colorado and lived in Denver; there were 344 such children.

Next came the identification of controls—344 healthy children of the same ages as the cases. These were chosen from Colorado birth certificates. Then came the task of evaluating the magnetic field exposures of each child in the study, both cases and controls. This was done by visiting each of the approximately 1000 homes in which these children had lived (many of the children had lived in more than one home) and making an assessment of exposure through application of the Wertheimer-Leeper wire code (see chapter 3).

After analyzing the data, the investigators concluded that living in a high-exposure home, as defined by the wiring code of the home (VHCC), increased the risk of childhood cancer on the order of twofold to threefold. The excess in risk was not limited to any one type of cancer.

The Reaction

The Wertheimer-Leeper study met with a good deal of skepticism in the scientific community. One reason was biological plausibility: if ambient power-frequency magnetic fields were producing biological effects, it was believed that the effects were due to electrical currents induced in tissues of the body. The magnitude of these induced currents can readily be calculated from widely available equations. Comparison of these calculated induced currents with those that occur spontaneously from natural electrical activity within the body shows that the increment produced by currents due to **ambient magnetic field**s is a fraction of 1% of those that occur naturally (Te89). Critics questioned how such a small increment in electric currents in the body (compared with those that occur naturally) could possibly produce serious biological consequences.

There was also considerable criticism of the method of exposure assessment—the wire coding. Some felt it unlikely that indoor exposures to EMF could be adequately assessed from wire codes, which were, after all, based on a crude visual assessment of neighboring power lines.

Another feature of the Wertheimer-Leeper study that provoked some criticism was the absence of "blinding." Because there always exists the possibility that a researcher may introduce bias while collecting data, it is highly desirable that the investigator not know whether the data pertain to a case or a control. In the Wertheimer-Leeper study, investigators knew whether the house they were examining was the home of a case or the home of a control.

Follow-up Studies

The year following the publication of the Wertheimer-Leeper study saw the publication of a study with a similar design, conducted in Rhode Island by Fulton, Cobb, and associates, that found no association between wire codes and childhood leukemia, (Fu80).

The Fulton study was criticized for the use of a control group quite different from the cases in terms of residential stability. Since families that move more frequently are likely to be different from families that are stable, and since these differences could also be related to the occurrence of leukemia, the use of such controls could introduce a bias (We80).

The Fulton study was followed by one conducted in Stockholm by Lennart Tomenius, a Swedish epidemiologist. It produced anomalous results: for exposures based on measurements of fields at the front door of the residence, it found an increase in the risk of brain cancer, but the study also found a reduction in leukemia risk among children living near power lines (To86).

The Savitz Study

Another landmark study was conducted by David Savitz, an epidemiologist then at the University of Colorado, now at the University of North Carolina. The Savitz study was one of the 16 studies undertaken by the New York Power Lines Project (see Chapter 1). The Scientific Advisory Committee to the Power Lines Project, aware of the Wertheimer-Leeper study, was interested in determining whether the results could be confirmed, and selected Savitz to examine the association between magnetic fields and childhood cancer.

Although this study also took place in Denver and in other ways was similar to that of Wertheimer-Leeper, there were some important differences. The Savitz cases were selected from a cancer registry rather than from death certificates, which meant that the diagnoses were more rigorously confirmed. In addition to assessing exposure by the use of the Wertheimer-Leeper code, Savitz and his colleagues also entered homes, where possible, for the purpose of making actual "spot" measurements of EMF in several rooms of the home. Another key difference was that the exposure assessment, the wire coding and the measurements of the homes, were carried out in a "blind" fashion, i.e., the investigators did not know whether the home was that of a case or a control.

Savitz's conclusions were similar to those of the Wertheimer-Leeper study, in that the cancer risk for children living in high-exposure homes, as estimated by the Wertheimer-Leeper code, was more than twice that for children living in homes with lower exposures. But the findings showed that measured fields were not so strongly associated with cancer risk as were the wire codes. The measured magnetic fields in the homes of children with cancer were only slightly different from those found in the homes of healthy children. There was no relationship between measured electric fields and cancer risk.

This apparent discrepancy in the results for the two means of assessing exposure (wire codes and direct measurements) created a dilemma: if the wire code is a surrogate for magnetic fields, the measured fields should show an association at least as strong or stronger than the surrogate.

How could these apparently anomalous findings be explained? Some people suggested that the apparent increase in the rate of cancer among children living near power lines was the result of some third factor, i.e., a confounder such as something found near power lines other than magnetic fields. Others suggested that it was indeed the magnetic fields producing the cancers, and that the wire codes were a more-accurate measure of long-term exposures than the spot measurements, i.e., the spot measurements may not be representative of long-term exposures.

The London Study (Lo91)

Given this background, there was a good deal of anticipation of the results of a study of EMF exposure conducted at the University of Southern California. This study, sponsored by the Electric Power Research Institute, had certain advantages over the earlier ones, particularly in that it used a newly developed exposure meter (EMDEX) that was left in place for 24 or more hours, and therefore captured considerably more exposure information than was possible with the earlier "spot" or instantaneous measurements used in the Savitz study. The

Table 9.2   Risk of Childhood Leukemia in Relation to 24-Hour Magnetic Field Measurements and Wertheimer–Leeper Wiring Configuration Class, Los Angeles, California, 1980–1987 (Lo 91)

	24–Hour Measurements (percentile)					
0-49	50–74		75–89		90–100	
	RR	95% CL	RR	95% CL	RR	95% CL
1.00	0.68	0.39–1.17	0.89	0.46–1.71	1.48	0.66–3.29
	Wiring Code					
Underground and Very Low	Ordinary Low		Ordinary High		Very High	
1.00	0.95	0.53–1.70	1.44	0.81–2.56	2.15	1.08–4.28

RR = Risk Ratio
CL = Confidence Limits

Wertheimer-Leeper wire codes were used as an additional method of exposure assessment, and spot measurements were made as well. The study examined over 240 cases of childhood leukemia.

Interestingly, the London study, instead of clarifying the issues, appears to have added to the mystery. No matter how data from the spot or 24-hour measurements are analyzed, there is no statistically significant relationship of the measured magnetic fields with leukemia (Lo 91). While the children living in the highest exposure category (mean exposure level greater than 2.7 mG) show a modest increase in risk (less than twofold), the finding is not statistically significant at the 95 percent confidence level. Further, the children living in the intermediate category homes (exposure level between .68 and 1.18 mG) appear to have a lower (but not statistically significant) risk than the children living in the lowest-exposure homes (less than .67 mG). As in the Savitz study, there was no relationship between measured electric fields and risk of leukemia.

On the other hand, when exposure to magnetic fields was measured through the use of wire codes comparable to that used by Wertheimer-Leeper, the result was similar to that found in both the Wertheimer-Leeper and Savitz studies, i.e., about a two to threefold increase in risk of leukemia among children living in the highest exposure category. Further, the exposure-risk relationship is statistically significant. That is, there is a significant trend in the relationship between exposure category and risk (Table 9.2).

The Feychting-Ahlbom Study

In 1992, another residential study of EMF exposure and cancer of both children and adults was completed. This study, conducted by Drs. Maria Feychting and Anders Ahlbom, was a case-control study of cancer occurrence among all persons living within 300 meters of transmission lines in Sweden during the period 1960–1985 (Fe93). Almost 500,000 persons satisfied these criteria. Cancers in this population were identified from the Swedish National Cancer Registry, in which cancers among Swedes are recorded upon diagnosis. All types of childhood cancers were examined, and in each case the EMF exposure was compared with that of four controls chosen from the same population. Among the adult population, only leukemia and brain cancer were studied (The adult results are described at the end of this chapter).

Four means of exposure assessment were used:

- Measured fields in the homes

- A computer model used to estimate historical fields

- Measured distance of the home to the lines

- In a few cases, 24-hour measurements of fields

The computer model involved consideration of the distance of the home to the lines, the configuration of the lines on the towers, and the amount of power being carried—factors that affect the magnetic field level in the house. Because historical annual power load data were available from the utilities, magnetic fields could be calculated for the year of particular interest, the year of the diagnosis for each case.

One hundred forty-one cases of childhood cancer were found in the population. Twelve of these were among children in the group calculated to have experienced residential field levels greater than 2 mG (which included approximately 10 percent of all homes). This was close to the number that might be expected if there were no effect from magnetic field exposure; the risk ratio using the calculated fields was 1.1 (Table 9.3).

For childhood leukemias alone, 38 cases were found, of which 7 were in children living in higher-exposure homes, i.e., above 2 mG. Compared with the controls, this produced a risk-ratio of almost three (2.7); that is, EMF exposure was associated with an almost threefold risk of leukemia. There was no effect on brain cancers.

Table 9.3   Risk of Childhood Cancer Among Children Living in Homes Above 2 mG (calculated)

	Total Number of Cases	Number of Cases > 2mG	RR(CL)
All cancers	141	12	1.1 (0.5–2.1)
Leukemia	38	7	2.7 (1.0–6.3)
Brain tumors	33	2	0.7 (0.1–2.7)

When exposures were estimated using measured fields, there was no association with any form of childhood cancer, including leukemia; this result is similar to that of the Savitz and London studies.

The study results, then, are similar in many ways to those of the previous studies, showing an increased risk of cancer among children when exposure is estimated by a model of power line fields, but not when fields are measured directly.

However, the study results also differ somewhat from those of previous studies in not showing an increased risk for cancers other than leukemias. In some of those other studies, brain cancer has been more consistently elevated than the leukemias. For example, in the Wertheimer-Leeper, Tomenius, and Savitz studies, the risk ratios for brain cancer were all 2 or greater. There is no obvious explanation for these differences.

An absence of an increase in brain cancer has also been found in a more recent study specifically directed to brain cancer in children, that conducted by Susan Preston-Martin of the University of Southern California (Pr94). Exposure assessment included both wire coding and measurments, as well as examination of EMF exposure to the parents. None of these measures of exposure showed a statistically significant association with brain cancer risk.

Other Studies

Denmark.   Another recent study examined residential EMF exposures of all children found in the Danish Tumor Registry with diagnoses of leukemia, brain tumor, or lymphoma in the period 1968–1986. The total number of cases was 1707. Exposures for these children and their controls were calculated on the basis of residential distance from transmission lines and known power load on the lines. The results showed no increase in leukemia or brain cancer, but a fivefold increase in the risk of lymphoma; however, this estimate was based on only three cases (Ol93). Such a small sample is inadequate one from which to draw conclusions.

Greece. A study of 170 cases of childhood leukemia in Greece, conducted by investigators collaborating with the Harvard School of Public Health, examined, among several factors, the possible effect of proximity to power lines. The study compared the risk of leukemia among children living close to power lines with that of children living at greater distances. No association was found (Pe93). Unfortunately, proximity of the child's residence to power lines was ascertained exclusively by the judgment of parents—no independent measurements were made.

Finland. Investigators from Helsinki University, the Finnish Cancer Registry, and the Finnish Power Company examined cancer cases among all children in Finland, comparing cancer rates among those living within 500 meters (about 550 yards) of power lines with rates among all Finnish children. Of the 135,000 children who had lived in the neighborhood of power lines during the years 1970–1989, there were 140 cases of cancer, compared with an expected number of 145. Thirty-five cases of leukemia were found (37 expected) (Ve93). The study, then, showed no evidence of cancer risk among children living near high voltage power lines.

Electrical Appliances and Cancer

As we have seen, wiring codes and household measurements of magnetic fields have both been used as surrogates for magnetic field exposures. Still another possible proxy for magnetic field exposures is the use of electrical appliances.

The London and Savitz studies both provided information about the use of electric appliances among the study subjects. Statistically significant associations of leukemia were found with the use of black-and-white television sets and electric hair dryers in the London study (Lo91) while the Savitz study shows a decreased risk (risk ratio 0.5) associated with the use of hair dryers (Sa90c). Whereas most appliances are used briefly, exposure to electric blankets continues for several hours each night. Both the Savitz and London studies show an increase in risk associated with use of electric blankets, but neither finding was statistically significant.

Interpreting the Results of the Residential Studies

Where does this leave us with respect to the residential studies? While some studies of childhood cancer and EMF show no association, at least four studies—Wertheimer-Leeper, Savitz, London, and Feychting—do show an association of wire codes and cancer, mainly leukemia. Yet, actual measurements of the magnetic fields fail to confirm the fields themselves as the factor responsible for the wire code/cancer association.

Four explanations have been offered for these puzzling positive findings. One is that the wire codes are a surrogate for something other than magnetic fields. There are no strong candidates for a possible confounding factor, to which Howard Wachtel refers as "factor x." He has suggested that there may be social factors associated with high wire code homes that might explain the wire code/cancer linkage. For example, renters are more likely to live in high wire code homes than owners. Renter families are also at greater risk of childhood cancer than are owner families (Pe 95).

A second possibility is that magnetic fields are indeed behind the wire code/cancer connection, but that our measurements of exposures are inadequate, Perhaps we have failed to measure the biologically important quality of these fields. For example, it has been suggested that while the average fields may not be important biologically, "spikes" or switching transients (the abrupt but transient surges of the magnetic field that accompany the switching on of power equipment, including household appliances) could produce a biological response. For these to explain the wire code/cancer association, switching transients would have to be more common around homes in the higher wire code categories. We do not know this to be the case.

It is also possible that measurements taken to date are a poorer surrogate of long-term average fields than are the wire codes. After all, measurements are only a snapshot in time. They reflect all of those sources within and outside the house that contribute to residential exposure levels, but those sources change with time as wiring, loading on the lines, and other factors change. If the wiring code is more stable than the magnetic field levels in a home, then the wiring code could be a better surrogate of past exposures than contemporaneous magnetic field measurements.

The third possibility is that some of the investigators have been the victims of an unintended bias in the design of their epidemiological study. The validity of case-control studies depends strongly on appropriate selection of controls. If, for some reason, these investigators had unwittingly selected control homes that did not adequately reflect the prevalence of high wire code homes in the general population, they would have found an apparent, but unreal, "excess" of high wire code homes among the cases, i.e., a selection bias would have operated.

How could this happen? In two of the studies under discussion here, the Savitz and the London studies, controls were selected by "random digit dialing." With this technique, telephone numbers are randomly selected, the numbers are dialed, and the people who answer are asked for certain information to determine their appropriateness to participate in the study. One obvious bias resulting from that technique is that controls will be selected only from those who have telephones, whereas the cases may have been representative of the entire population (This is not true of the London study where the *cases* were required to have had telephones). While this possible bias may not be of much significance, a more important possible source of bias is the participation rate among the persons telephoned. If those who choose to participate are in some way different from non-participants, such differences could bias the outcome of the study.

Philip Cole, an epidemiologist at the University of Alabama, Birmingham, and Tom Jones, an engineer at the American Electric Power Company, have together suggested another possible source of bias in the wire coding studies. They point out that in the Savitz study, controls were required to have had residential stability (to have remained in the same home over a long period of time), whereas that condition was not required of the cases. They speculate that residential stability might be associated with wire codes, for example, that people living in "low wire code homes" might be more stable than people in "high wire code" homes. This theory was tested in a study carried out in Columbus, Ohio, and indeed, the hypothesis appeared to be corroborated (Jo93). To what extent this bias may have affected the outcome of the Savitz study is unknown. (In the USC study, this possible bias was investigated and found not to be a problem).

A British group of scientists who reviewed the epidemiological studies related to EMF exposure also found evidence of bias in the Savitz study (NRPB92). Put simply, their thesis is as follows: it appears that the children of low-income families have an increased risk of leukemia. Such families are also more likely to live near high-voltage power lines. However, there appeared to be too few low-income families among the controls. Thus, income could quite possibly be operating as a confounding factor. The group concluded, "These observations throw doubt on the overall validity of the study."

This possible bias was avoided in the Swedish (Fe93) study where controls were selected from the same population as the cases, that is, from those living within 300 meters of the transmission line.

All of these three possible explanations (inadequate measurement of magnetic fields, confounding, and bias) are now being tested in new studies specifically designed to examine these possibilities. For example, epidemiological studies of childhood leukemia utilizing portable exposure meters will provide improved measurements of exposures to children.

Wire code methodology is being improved, and studies of the characteristics of families in different wire code categories will tell us more about possible biases in epidemiological studies of power lines and cancer.

The fourth and final possible explanation of the assocations found in some studies is that they simply represent variability in small numbers. Childhood cancer is a rare disease, and all of the studies are necessarily limited in their statistical power. Such an explanation could account for the mixture of positive associations found together with negative studies, and the inconsistency in cancer types found.

Temporal Trends

Before leaving the subject of childhood cancer, we should consider a commonly stated objection to the EMF-childhood cancer association. The argument is that if electricity produces childhood cancer, then with the tremendous increase in electricity production and consumption over the past fifty years, we should be seeing an epidemic of childhood cancer. Since we do not, the argument goes, the association cannot be causal. That argument has been made most forcefully by John David Jackson, a professor of electrical engineering at the University of California, Berkeley (Ja92). In contrast, a Canadian research group has reported that they do find a correlation between childhood cancers (brain and leukemia) and the differing consumption of electrical energy among Canadian provinces (Kr94).

The problem with studies which examine the relationship between electrical power consumption and disease is that we have no data on the relationship between power consumption and exposure to EMF. While it may appear reasonable that EMF exposures rise in parallel with electricity consumption, we have no data on this relationship. Over the years, there have been too many changes in transmission design, household wiring, residential housing patterns, and appliance use to have any certainty about average exposure levels; it is even possible that some individual exposures have declined. Regional differences in these variables, as well as differences in medical care, also make studies such as the Canadian study, difficult to interpret.

Furthermore, data on the frequency of childhood cancer over long periods of time which would be necesary to an examination of temporal trends, are limited.

Lastly, an examination of temporal trends would be meaningful only if EMF were postulated to be the dominant cause of childhood cancer; most experts agree that if EMF is carcinogenic, it accounts for only a small percent of the disease. A minor cause of any disease could operate in different directions than other causes of the disease, obscuring the effects of a minor causal factor.

Adult Residential Studies

Wire coding as a means of assessing magnetic field exposure has also been used to study residential exposure and cancer among adults. Following their study of childhood cancer in children in Denver using the wire code methodology as a means of assessing exposure, Wertheimer-Leeper applied the same methodology to an examination of adult cancer in Denver and its suburbs. They concluded that an association existed between magnetic fields and cancers of the nervous system, uterus, breast, and lymph nodes (We82). Four subsequent studies have failed to find such an association (McD86, Se88, Co89, Yo91).

In the Swedish study of persons living near transmission lines cited above (Fe93), leukemias and brain cancers were examined in the adult population. There was no increase in total leukemias among those living in homes with magnetic field exposures calculated to be greater than 2 mG, but there was an increased risk for one subcategory of leukemia, chronic myelogenous leukemia. Howev-

Table 9.4 Risk of Leukemia and Brain Cancer Among Adults Living in Homes Above 2mG (calculated)

	Total Number of Cases	Number of Cases > 2mG	RR(CL)
All leukemia	284	17	1.6 (0.9–2.9)
Acute myeloid	63	5	2.1 (0.7–5.3)
Chronic myeloid	49	5	2.9 (1.0–7.3)
Brain tumors	195	4	0.5 (0.2–1.4)

*Exposures calculated ten years prior to diagnosis.

er, there was a decreased risk for another subgroup, lymphatic leukemia, among the most highly exposed population (Table 9.4).

A subsequent study of a Dutch population of more than 1500 persons who had lived below a transmission line where indoor magnetic fields were 1.0 to 11.0 mG for at least five years showed no evidence of an increase in mortality; however, the number of cases was too small to reach any conclusions about individual causes of death (Sc93).

Cancer and Electric Blanket Use in Adults

Because electric blankets increase EMF exposure significantly (in the order of 10–15 mG) and for considerable periods of time, and because exposure is relatively easy to ascertain just by asking – the association of electric blanket use and cancer has been investigated. There are two published reports of electric blanket use and leukemia in adults (Se88, Pr93); there is also a single study of breast cancer (Ve91) and testicular cancer (Ve90) among electric blanket users. None of these showed any increased risk as a result of electric blanket use.

An Overview of the Residential Studies

In Chapter 8, it was suggested that certain criteria are helpful in assessing the strength of epidemiological evidence related to assessing the health effects of a putative environmental agent. In the following, the relevant criteria are applied to the residential EMF evidence reviewed in this chapter:

Magnitude of Risk and Precision.   If one focuses only on the four studies of childhood cancer that utilized wire coding for exposure assessment (Wertheimer-Leeper, Savitz, London, Feychting), the risk was increased by a factor of 2 to 3 for those in the highest exposure category. To some epidemiologists, this level of increased risk is close to the "noise level." Studies utilizing residential magnetic field measurements show smaller and insignificant associations with cancer.

The studies of adult cancer and residential exposures to EMF for the most part show no association.

Exposure-Response Relationship. All four studies of childhood cancer that used wire codes show a slight trend of increased risk with increased exposure as measured by wire codes. The trend does not exist when exposure is assessed by field measurements.

Among adults, the Feychting study showed an exposure-response relationship only for one subgroup of leukemias, the acute myelogenous leukemias.

Exposure Assessment. As repeatedly emphasized here, exposure assessment of EMF has a double problem—ignorance of the biologically relevant parameter of those fields, and the difficulty of reconstructing past exposures. One consequence of these difficulties in exposure assessment could be an underestimate of risk; that is, if we better understood biologically significant parameters of exposure, risk estimates could be higher than currently estimated by our crude measures of exposure. It is also possible that with such knowledge, risks of exposure could disappear entirely.

Consistency. A disturbing observation about both the childhood and the adult studies is the inconsistency with respect to the diseases found. The two Denver studies found an increase in risk for all childhood cancers, possibly greater for brain cancer than for leukemia; one Swedish study found no significant increase in childhood brain cancer but an increase in leukemia (Fe92), while another Swedish study found an increase of brain cancer, but a decreased risk of leukemia (To86). To most observers and reviewers, there is no adequate explanation for these inconsistencies other than the possibility that we are simply observing random variability.

Among adults, the Feychting study reports an increase in chronic myelogenous leukemias, but other studies have shown a greater effect among the acute leukemias.

Consistency, like beauty, is in the eye of the beholder. While many observers find inconsistency among the childhood cancer studies, Ahlbom and Feychting find a good deal of consistency. They dismiss the Tomenius study, which found reduced leukemia risk, on the basis of questionable exposure assessment. They also point out that, including their own study, there are six studies that find an excess risk of childhood leukemia and some measure of EMF (Ah93a)

There are also many studies that find no increase in cancer at all. Several studies have been described here, including those conducted in Rhode Island (Fu80), Greece (Pe93), Finland (Ko93), and southern California (Pr94), that show no evidence of an increase in cancer risk among children living near power lines. Other negative studies from Taiwan (Li89) and England (Co89, My85) have also been reported.

Summary

Epidemiological studies of cancer in populations exposed to sources of EMF in the home have been reviewed. While some studies have been described that report an increased risk of cancer in exposed populations among children, the studies of cancer among adults living in high magnetic field homes have not, as a whole, shown such a relationship.

It has been noted that the type of cancer found in exposed populations is inconsistent, the risk sometimes being found in brain cancer, in other studies leukemia, although the type of leukemia found has also been inconsistent.

Beginning with the relatively crude assessment of exposure utilized in the initial study of Wertheimer-Leeper in 1979, subsequent studies have attempted to resolve the uncertain nature of the relationship between exposure and cancer risk by utilizing increasingly sophisticated measures of exposure. In spite of those improvements in exposure assessment, in some studies the risk of certain cancers has remained in the range of a factor of two; many studies find no risk at all. Generally, the risks found using distance from power lines (as a measure of magnetic field exposure) have been greater than when direct measurements of magnetic fields have been utilized.

Four possible explanations have been offered for the discrepancy in the risk found with the two measures of EMF exposure (direct and indirect) utilized in these studies: inadequate measurement of magnetic fields, the existence of confounding factors, bias in the conduct of the studies, and random variability in small numbers.

10

Occupational Studies: EMF and Cancer

Epidemiological studies of working populations serve two functions: they provide information about the safety of the working environment, and they alert us to hazards from high exposures to agents in the workplace which may help identify hazards to the general population. Much of our early knowledge of environmental hazards comes from studies of the health of working populations.

As a consequence, a large number of studies of persons working in **electrical occupations** have been conducted for the purpose of evaluating possible carcinogenic effects of EMF.

Exposure Assessment in Occupational Studies

A variety of means have been used to characterize the EMF exposures to persons in the workplace. Methods vary from those which are crude, but easily available, to those which are precise, but expensive and time consuming. These can be considered on a hierarchical

119

basis, from those which are crude and exploratory, to the most sophisticated and reliable:

1. Studies of employees of an industry or workplace where workers are assumed to be exposed to EMF. For example, cancer rates
   of persons in the utility industry might be compared with workers in an industry not likely to receive high exposures to EMF.
   An excess of cancer could be taken as suggestive of an EMF effect. The weakness of such studies are the aggregation of all
   workers in an industry from clerks and managers with those
   most likely to be exposed, as well as the difficulty of adjusting
   for other possible factors that might influence cancer in the two
   or more industries under study.

2. Studies of persons having the same job title, as described in
   Chapter 3, have been the most commonly used surrogate for exposure. While this data is easily available, it too is crude, in that it
   implies that exposures can be estimated from the title of the job
   alone, and that all persons in the same job category are equally
   exposed. This is clearly not the case, since work practices vary
   considerably within the job category. For example, electricians
   as a group vary enormously with respect to the amount of exposure that individual electricians may encounter, depending
   upon the various tasks that they may perform.

3. Measurements of EMF in the workplace may be utilized in epidemiological studies. While this is an improvement, individual
   workers may vary considerably in time spent in these environments, and exposures may vary considerably within the designated work space, i.e., the measurements may not be taken
   where workers spend most of their time. Here too there may be
   considerable variation among workers. Consider a study of
   EMF exposure among cooks. Where should the measurements
   be taken? How many kitchens must we measure? Not only do
   kitchens differ with respect to dimensions and equipment, but
   different cooks may have very different work practices.

4. Finally, with the use of personal exposure meters, which may be
   worn on a belt or carried in a shirt pocket, individual exposures
   may be recorded over a period of hours or days. Because these
   measurements are expensive, only a sample of workers can be
   measured, and only during a sample of the tasks performed.

Studies utilizing personal measurements are of the highest validity in establishing a link between exposure and disease.

In general, measurements of EMF show that workers in electrical occupations such as substation workers and electricians do have EMF exposures higher than those of other workers, but these vary greatly among persons with the same job title, and among those with various job titles. Average exposures vary from those found in the usual office environment to average exposures at the high end of about ten mG with peak exposures of thousands of mG (EPRI94).

Finally, occupational exposure assessment suffers from the same problem bedeviling residential exposure assessment, namely, that we cannot be certain of just which parameter of exposure is important to measure—the average exposure throughout the workday, the highest exposures, or some other characteristic.

While increased risks for a variety of cancers (e.g., melanoma, prostate) have been reported in excess in a small number of studies, the discussion here will be limited to cancers that have received the most research attention—leukemia, brain cancer, and breast cancer. Studies investigating cancer among the children of "electrical workers" will be addressed in the chapter on reproductive effects (Chapter 13).

Wertheimer-Leeper

The same report in which the results of the Wertheimer-Leeper childhood cancer study were published also included a brief examination of cancer among persons in electrical occupations (We79). While the information was quite limited, the authors concluded that cancer risks among persons in certain electrical occupations, such as linemen and substation workers, were increased by 15%. The authors concluded that "the harmlessness of EMF could not be proven" (the reader is reminded that harmlessness can never be proven). This first published report of cancer mortality among electrical workers has led to a considerable number of studies of cancer in workers presumed to be exposed to EMF—studies to be reviewed in this chapter.

Leukemias Among Electrical Workers

A follow-up study of cancer among electrical workers was conducted by Sam Milham, an epidemiologist working with the Washington State Health Department. As did Wertheimer and Leeper, Milham utilized job titles (see Chapter 3) as a means of assessing EMF exposure. The 11 different "electrical occupations" that he inferred might subject workers to high levels of EMF included such jobs as electricians, welders, power station operators, electronics assemblers, and motion picture projectionists (Mi85). Using death certificates, he reported an increased percentage of deaths due to leukemia among workers in these occupations, as compared with all other deaths.

Subsequent studies utilizing actual spot measurements of EMF exposure among members of various electrical occupations have shown that Milham's intuition about exposure among those electrical trades was good; workers in those jobs do, on the average, have higher exposures than do those in other job categories. Nevertheless, there is considerable variation of exposure within a single job category, and job titles remain a poor surrogate for epidemiological purposes (Chapter 3).

We now have a large number of studies of leukemia among electrical workers. George Hutchison, emeritus professor of epidemiology at Harvard University, analyzed data from 24 of these studies (Hu92). For all electrical job categories, the risk of death from leukemia was 19% greater than in non-electrical workers (risk ratio 1.19 [1.12 – 1.26]). In studies that reported the particular type of leukemia, it was the acute leukemias that were most often increased.

Table 10.1 shows the data arranged by particular occupational category. The highest risk is found among electrical equipment assemblers who have an risk ratio of 2.81 (1.64 – 4.84), whereas electricians have only a slightly elevated risk of 1.19 (1.04 – 1.36). In the studies considered by Hutchison to be among the better studies, the highest risk was among television and radio repairmen, with a risk ratio of 4.02 (2.01 – 8.04).

A recent study of cancer among the entire worker population of Norway appears to support an increased risk of leukemia among electrical workers (Ty92). In this study, 37,945 men were chosen whose jobs involved some degree of exposure to EMF. The investigators stratified the jobs into those with estimates of heavy, intermediate, and weak magnetic fields (no measurements were made). Those who were considered exposed to radio-frequency electric and magnetic fields were considered separately. Leukemia risks were highest among those exposed to radio frequencies (risk ratio 2.85). The risk

Table 10.1 Leukemia Risk by Occupation

	All Studies	Preferred Studies
1. Electrical equipment assemblers	2.81 (1.64, 4.84)	
2. Aluminum workers	1.78 (1.26, 2.51)	1.60 (0.82, 2.80)
3. Telegraph, radio. radar operators	1.59 (1.29, 1.96)	1.44 (1.10, 1.89)
4. Streetcar, subway, elevated railway motormen	1.43 (0.54, 3.81)	No Data
5. Power station operators	1.46 (1.01, 2.11)	1.16 (0.75, 1.79)
6. Electronic technicians	1.18 (0.75, 1.88)	1.01 (0.54, 1.88)
7. Power and telephone linemen	1.35 (1.06, 1.73)	1.22 (0.87, 1.71)
8. Electrical and electronic engineers	1.24 (1.05, 1.47)	1.19 (0.99, 1.43)
9. Electricians	1.19 (1.04, 1.36)	1.05 (0.88, 1.26)
10. Motion picture projectionists	1.53 (0.73, 3.21)	0.91 (0.23, 3.67)
11. Telephone repairers, installers	0.99 (0.70, 1.40)	
12. Welders, flame cutters	1.04 (0.80, 1.34)	1.01 (0.64, 1.58)
13. Television, radio repairmen	2.24 (1.37, 3.66)	4.02 (2.01, 8.04)
14. Coal miners	2.53 (1.12, 5.74)	
15. Electical, electronic fitters	1.44 (0.97, 2.15)	
16. Electric machine operators	1.08 (0.03, 5.90)	
17. Telephone operators	1.03 (0.60, 1.80)	
18. Radio, radar mechanics	0.47 (0.18, 1.26)	
All occupations	1.19 (1.12, 1.26)	1.11 (1.03, 1.20)

of leukemia (and the confidence levels) among those exposed to EMF was as follows:

Heavy magnetic	1.79 (1.09–2.76)
Intermediate magnetic	1.36 (0.81–2.16)
Weak magnetic	1.10 (0.70–1.63)
Weak electric and magnetic	0.92 (0.19–2.70)

The increasing risk with increasing exposure lends support to an association between EMF exposure and leukemia.

The Floderus Study of Swedish Workers (Fl93)

Recently, results of a Swedish occupational study of leukemia and EMF, conducted by Brigitta Floderus and colleagues in the Swedish National Institute of Occupational Health have become available. All leukemias and brain cancers occurring in men living in central Sweden were identified from the National Cancer Registry for the years 1983–1987. There were 250 leukemias found. Two controls were chosen from the Swedish national census for each case. The occupations of cases and controls were identified from the written questionnaire sent to study subjects or their families.

Spot measurements were made with exposure meters for workers in each of 168 different job categories. The exposures were divided into quartiles and risk ratios were calculated for each quartile. The exposures for the highest quartile were 2.9 mG and above. For all leukemias, there was a statistically significant risk ratio for the highest exposure category (risk ratio 1.6 [1.07 – 2.37]). For the 107 cases of chronic lymphatic leukemia, there was a risk ratio of 3.04 (1.58 – 5.84) in the highest EMF exposure category.

Although the Floderus study provided better estimates of exposure than previous occupational studies, not all reviewers agree with its conclusions. The Oak Ridge Associated Universities panel has raised significant questions about the validity of the study results, citing differences in the treatment of cases and controls, low rate of cooperation among the cases and controls, and poor exposure assessment (OR93). Still, the study set a new standard for occupational studies of EMF substituting measurements for job titles.

Studies of Electrical Utility Workers

Three studies of cancer, including leukemia, have been completed among the employees of large electric utilities. In all of these studies, spot measurements were made of magnetic fields experienced by workers in different jobs within the company. On the basis of those measurements, exposures were then assigned to each study participant, aggregating both level of exposure and years of exposure.

The first of these studies was conducted by Jack Sahl and co-workers, who examined mortality among more than 36,000 employees, both active and retired, of the Southern California Edison Company. In comparing "electrical" workers with non-electrical workers (the distinction was made on the basis of careful measurements of exposures), they found no evidence of an increased risk of any cancer, including leukemia, in this worker population (Sa93b).

A similar study was conducted among employees of three large utility systems in Canada and France (Th94). The study differed from the one in southern California in being a study of cancer incidence rather than cancer mortality. While there was no increase in cancer as a whole, there was a statistically significant increase in acute leukemia, especially of the myeloid variety (risk ratio 3.2 [1.2–8.3]); however, there was no exposure-response trend. This finding contrasted with the Floderus study, where an increased risk was found for chronic lymphatic leukemia.

Finally, a study of the mortality of almost 140,000 employees of five large U.S. utility was conducted by David Savitz and Dana Loomis (Sa95). The study examined the death certificates of these men, of which there were more than 20,000. Exposure was assesssed in a number of ways; no increase in leukemia was found.

Leukemia Among Welders

Studies of leukemia among welders are of particular interest. Welders are exposed to very high fields, to so-called "transients," and to fields that vary widely throughout the day as the welding torch is switched on and off. Average exposures during arc welding are in the order of a thousand mG, and reach several thousand mG at the maximum (St89). Because of concern about cancer in these workers who are also constantly exposed to metal and other fumes, many epidemiological studies of welders have been conducted, including studies of leukemia. A British committee of scientists and epidemiologists recently completed a review of 15 different studies of leukemia among welders (NRPB92). The results of these individual studies are shown in Table 10.2. Studies in the upper part of the table are specifically of welders, whereas those in the lower part are studies in which welders were but one of many groups of electrical workers studied. The total number of leukemia cases expected was 198.55; the observed number was 187. (In all cases, the expected number of cases was calculated from the number of cases of leukemia found among non-electrical workers.)

The absence of an excess of leukemia and the consistency of the results among the studies can be interpreted as evidence that EMF exposures in the working environment of welders are not a significant cause of leukemia.

Brain Cancer

While the possibility of an increased risk of leukemia as a result of exposure to EMF has been the main focus of research attention, brain cancer among electrical workers has also been studied.

Table 10.2   Risk Ratios For Leukemia in Various Studies of Welders

Study	Observed	Expected	Risk Ratio
Calle and Savitz	20	25.30	0.8
Gallagher et al	8	8.89	0.9
Juutilainen et al	5	5.00	1.0
Milham	19	21.30	0.9
Office of Population Censuses and Surveys	19	20.65	1.0
Polednak	0	1.56	0.0
Stern et al	7	3.10	2.3
Törnqvist et al	39	39.00	1.0
Working Group	6	9.49	0.6
Wright et al	6	6.24	1.0
Becker et al	0	1.20	0.0
Puntoni et al	15	13.20	1.1
Sjögren and Carstensen	43	43.62	1.0
Subtotal	58	58.02	1.0

Some 17,500 new cases of brain cancer occur in the United States each year —1.5 % of all cancers (Ca94).

Leukemias are relatively easy to diagnose, since samples of blood, from which the diagnosis is usually made, are easily available. In contrast, brain tumors are not easily diagnosed, and can be easily confused with other diseases affecting the brain, including metastases from cancers elsewhere in the body, thereby leading to erroneous diagnoses of brain cancer whereas in fact the cancer is in the lung or abdomen. However, the development of new scanning techniques has improved the diagnosis of brain tumors. This has been speculated to be at least part of the explanation for a recent increase in the reported incidence of brain cancer.

There is considerable uncertainty about the causes of brain cancer. Perhaps the best-characterized cause is ionizing radiation: We now know that radiation of the scalp of children with ringworm is followed by an increase in all types of brain cancer (Ro88).

A variety of occupations have been tentatively associated with an increased risk of brain cancer. These include the petrochemical industry, the rubber industry, agriculture, the nuclear industry, and certain white-collar occupations (Ro91a).

An early study of brain cancer among electrical workers was carried out by Ruey Lin, working at the Maryland State Department of Health. Using death certificates, he was able to identify the occupations of electrical workers and a group of controls (Li85). To estimate EMF exposure, he asked a panel of experts to rank exposure in these

Table 10.3   Risk Ratios For Brain Cancer Among Adults With Occupational Exposure to EMF, Various Studies

Reference	Risk Ratios (95% Confidence Limits)
Lin 1987	4.10 (2.49, 7.42)
Törnqvist 1986	1.17 (0.79, 1.70)
Gubéran 1989	1.54 (0.13, 9.14)
Milham 1985	1.23 (0.99, 1.48)
Milham 1988	1.39 (0.93, 2.04)
Loomis 1989	1.50 (1.00, 2.10)
Preston-Martin 1989	1.80 (0.70, 4.80)
McLaughlin 1987	0.90 (0.69, 1.16)
Lin 1985	1.57 (1.19, 2.06)
Thomas 1987	1.60 (1.00, 2.40)
Speers 1988	1.39 (0.93, 2.07)
Reif 1989	0.79 (0.39, 1.59)
Lewis 1990	0.65 (0.40, 1.09)
Olin 1985	1.00 (0.10, 3.70)
Vågerö 1985	1.00 (0.30, 2.30)
Magnani 1987	1.30 (0.70, 2.50)

Summary odds ratio 1.24 (1.12, 1.36)

occupations as definite, probable, possible, or none. Risk ratios and confidence limits for these categories follow:

Definite exposure	2.15 (1.10 – 4.06)
Probable exposure	1.95 (0.94 – 3.91)
Possible exposure	1.44 (1.06 – 1.95)
No exposure	1.00

A similar study also found an elevated risk ratio for brain cancer in the "definite exposure" category (1.6), but not other categories (Le90).

A review of studies of brain cancer among electrical occupations has recently been completed (Hu92). These studies, together with the risk ratios found in each, are shown in Table 10.3. One is always tempted to aggregate studies such as those in this series, adding their results; however, individual studies differ considerably from each other in the range of occupations studied, the means of exposure assessment, and the sample sizes, among other factors. Nevertheless, Hutchison has carefully aggregated the studies and finds a summary risk ratio of 1.24 (1.12–1.36).

Since the Hutchison review, additional studies of brain cancer in electrical workers have been completed. The Floderus study described above also examined brain cancer and EMF exposure. For most of the analyses conducted, there was a small increase in risk (about 1.5) in the highest exposure category, the precise risk depending upon which of the measures of magnetic field was used. As the investigators summarized the situation, "Some results speak in favor of an association" (Fl93).

The three studies of utility workers cited above also investigated brain cancer among electrical workers. The Sahl study showed no evidence of an increased risk of this disease (Sa93b), whereas a second study showed an increased risk of one particular type of brain cancer (astrocytoma), but the numbers were small and the authors conclude that the association is "more likely artificial than real" (Th94). In contrast, the Savitz study did suggest an increase in brain cancer, with a risk ratio of 2.6 in the highest exposure category. The weakness of this latter observation is that the observation was limited to death certificate diagnoses, and were not confirmed by clinical data.

Breast Cancer

Breast cancer is rare among men, occurring at a rate about 100 times lower than that found among women. In the United States, male breast cancer occurs at a rate of less than 1:100,000 persons per year—about 1,000 cases per year (Ca94). It is most common in the real estate, newspaper, and health care industries, and among government workers (Th93). When it does occur, it can be a very malignant and rapidly progressing form of cancer.

Genevieve Matanoski, an epidemiologist at the Johns Hopkins School of Public Health, was studying health records of New York Telephone Company employees when she unexpectedly found two cases of male breast cancer in a population of 50,582 men, among whom only 0.3 cases would have been expected (Ma91b). The risk ratio was 6.5 (0.79–23.5). The remarkable thing was that both of these cases were found among men who had the same job—providing maintenance on switching equipment, where there may have been increased exposures to switching transients (brief surges in EMF). This observation first raised the question of EMF and breast cancer, as well as the question of whether switching transients could be an important factor in EMF exposures, a question to which some current research is being directed.

Little is known about the causes of male breast cancer, so Matanoski's report has attracted a good deal of interest, not only because of the possible implications for male breast cancer, but also because it could possibly be a clue to the much more common cancer of the female breast.

Epidemiologist Paul Demers and co-workers at the University of Washington carried out a case-control study of 227 male breast cancer cases in which they examined the occupations of these men (De90). They found an overall risk ratio for breast cancer for any job presumably exposed to high levels of EMF of 1.8 (1.0–3.2). For certain specific groups of workers—electricians, telephone linemen, and electrical power workers—the risk ratio for breast cancer was 6.0 (1.7–21.5).

A Scandinavian study supports an increased risk of breast cancer among men presumably exposed to EMF (Ty92). In this study, among the 37,952 men in electrical occupations (e.g., railroad employees, power plant employees, radio repairmen), 12 cases of breast cancer were found, whereas only 5.8 would be expected.

While such risk increases appear to be impressive, these studies suffer from the absence of adequate exposure assessment; we do not know with any certainty that the men who developed breast cancer were exposed to higher levels of EMF than others. Further, there have also been studies that *failed* to show any increase in risk of breast cancer among persons presumed to be exposed to EMF occupationally (Ro94) or from electric blanket use (Ve91).

Among women, breast cancer is the most common cancer, and any hints of possible causal factors, such as EMF, justify careful study in women, particularly since known risk factors appear to be similar for both male and female breast cancer (ionizing radiation, family history). The highest risk found by Wertheimer and Leeper in their study of residential EMF and cancer in adults was for the female breast (We87). Loomis, Savitz and Ananth searched the death certificates of women in 24 states to identify almost 28,000 women who had died of breast cancer. They compared the risks of this disease among electrical occupations (as indicated on the death certificate) with breast cancer among women in non-electrical occupations. They found a 40 percent increase in breast cancer among these women, highest among electrical engineers (Lo94). In an editorial accompanying the article, Trichopoulos cites 6 studies in which no association between EMF exposure and female breast cancer were found (Tr94).

Breast cancer is increasing among women in industrialized nations. What do industrialized nations have that non-industrialized nations do not have? Two possible factors are more dietary fat and changes in patterns of reproduction. It has also been noted that an increased use of electricity and illumination are associated with industrialization; they are being studied as possible causes of breast cancer (St92a).

SUMMARY

In this chapter, studies of cancer among persons occupationally exposed to EMF have been reviewed. Attention has been focused particularly on leukemia, brain cancer, and breast cancer.

Early studies were conducted with job titles as the means of exposure assessment. Those studies, while inconsistent, generally showed risk ratios in the order of 1.2 for both leukemia and brain cancer. Breast cancer has only recently come under investigation.

For exposure assessment, more recent studies have utilized measurements of magnetic fields in the workplace. Nevertheless, the association between EMF exposure and cancer remains problematic. Particularly troubling is the inconsistency among studies, some showing a modest increase in leukemia, but not brain cancer, while others show the opposite, or nothing at all.

Most reviewers of the EMF occupational epidemiology consider the evidence of causation weak. For example, the Advisory Committee to the British National Radiation Protection Board headed by Sir Richard Doll concludes as follows:

"The many investigations into the possibility of an occupational hazard of cancer from exposure to extremely low frequency electromagnetic fields have not provided any evidence of a quantitative relationship between risk and level of exposure. The very small excess risk of leukemia in the total database may be attributed to selection bias in favor of the publication of positive results. The greater excess of brain cancer may indicate an occupational hazard from some types of electronic work but the nature of the hazard (if it exists) is unclear. No conclusion can be drawn from the reports of excesses of other types of cancer, but the experimental evidence justifies further investigation of an occupational hazard of breast cancer in men" (NRPB92).

11

Disease Clusters

Reports of clusters of cancer and other diseases resulting from exposures to EMF are increasingly common in the press. Some examples:

An alleged cluster of cancer cases in the upscale San Francisco suburb of Mill Valley, California, said to be the result of exposure to EMF, gave rise to a newspaper magazine section cover article entitled "Poison in Paradise" (Wh93b).

In the *New Yorker* magazine and in his two books, Paul Brodeur has cited several examples of alleged clusters of disease near sources of EMF such as power lines and electrical substations (Br89, Br93b).

Do these clusters tell us something significant about the role of EMF in causing disease, or do they represent nothing more than the operation of chance? Are they true clusters? What is a true cluster? Chance can certainly play tricks; if a cluster is defined as an occurrence of cases that would not happen more than once in a hundred times, then, in a large state with many hundreds of communities and with many diseases that might attract attention, dozens of clusters will occur each year, whether recognized or not.

The problem is something like throwing a handful of beans onto a checkerboard: some squares will be covered with very few beans, or none at all, while many others will have more than the average number—they are clusters, occurring purely by chance.

How does the epidemiologist determine which of the many reported clusters of disease represent the result of environmental exposures, and which are only chance collections of cases? There are actually two issues: the first is the determination of whether the alleged cluster is a true cluster, that is, whether the cases have been collected in a valid manner and the number of cases found is truly statistically significant, i.e., unlikely to have occurred by chance alone. If a cluster is confirmed, then the second question arises: is this cluster the result of some identifiable environmental exposure? There always remains the possibility that the cluster occurred as a matter of chance—just as drawing a royal flush in poker is a rare event, but does in fact occur.

The following diagram represents the process of investigating a reported cluster. Step 1 is the determination of the existence of a cluster, Step 2 is the determination of the cause—chance (no obvious explanation) or demonstrable cause (real).

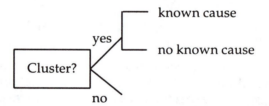

It is to be emphasised that the absence of a statistically significant cluster does not necessarily exclude the operation of a weak environmental cause. It does mean an environmental cause becomes unlikely.

Cluster: A Definition

A disease cluster is defined by the Centers for Disease Control as "an unusual aggregation of health events, real or perceived." Generally, a cluster refers to an unexpectedly high number of cases in a geographic area or worker population within a given period of time, i.e., there are both time and space characteristics. To illustrate, consider a small city, let us call it Middletown, in which five cases of a given disease, on average, would be expected to occur each year if the rates for this size population were the same as those for the state as a whole. The following pattern is noted:

Year	Number of cases
1979	2
1980	3
1981	8
1982	10
1983	9
1984	3
1985	0

In the year 1984, a cluster is reported to the Middletown Health Department—27 cases over the previous three years, whereas only 15 cases would be expected within a 3-year period. But, if one examines the entire 7-year experience, there are thirty-five cases, exactly as one would expect on the basis of state-wide rates. The point is that a cluster will have both *time* and *space* characteristics, and that arbitrary selection of the boundaries of either can lead to the creation of an apparent cluster.

Clusters may come to attention as the result of routine and systematic observation of data, i.e., a determined search for aggregations of cases. For example, the National Cancer Institute has constructed maps of cancer occurrence throughout the United States, looking for clusters that might provide clues to cause of certain cancers.

Or, clusters may be identified as the result of concern on the part of members of a population who experience, or think they are experiencing, an excess of disease.

The difficulty with this informal process is that clusters can be created by arbitrarily establishing boundaries, in either time or space, for the cluster. Those boundaries can be selected, whether consciously or unconsciously, to create a cluster where none exists. In the above case of Middletown, selecting the years 1983–1985, and ignoring the preceding and subsequent years, would create a cluster—a process of arbitrarily selecting boundaries of time or space that has come to be known as the Texas Sharpshooter Phenomenon.

The Texas Sharpshooter Phenomenon

Briefly, this sharpshooter first fires several bullets at a barn door, after which he paints a bull's eye around the bullet holes. This situation
is equivalent to a resident of a community who becomes concerned
about a particular disease, often cancer, and begins to collect similar
cases among neighbors in nearby homes, whether living there now
or in the past. This is particularly likely to happen if there is a source
of pollution nearby which has raised health concerns in the neighborhood.

The problem with this procedure is that discoverers of such clusters often paint the bull's eye after counting cases. That is, the boundaries of the area where the cluster apparently occurs are chosen to fit
the area where the excess of cases has already been identified—
whether on the same neighborhood block or community. A few cases
of a rare disease occurring in one block may appear to be a great excess but if the entire community is surveyed, the number of cases is
no greater than what would be expected on the basis of chance
alone—something like the excess number of beans falling on the
same square of the checkerboard.

Here is an illustration of the Sharpshooter Phenomenon: members
of the epidemiology group of the National Cancer Institute set out to
investigate whether clusters of childhood leukemia exist in Los Angeles. They wanted to know whether there were geographic clusters
that might provide clues as to causation. They first examined the frequency of childhood leukemias among all of the 32 regions of the
county. The numbers of cases varied among those regions —some regions rather high and some low, just as would be expected if beans
had been thrown on the map of Los Angeles. However, when the investigators marked a map with the residence of each case, they could
"create" four leukemia "clusters" by visually grouping cases across
region boundaries (Figure 11.I). They had illustrated the Texas
Sharpshooter Phenomenon—first find a cluster and then draw the
boundary around it (Gl68)

Although epidemiologists and health officers would very much
prefer that the identification of clusters result from systematic examination of data, as in the Los Angeles study of leukemia by census
tract cited above, they nevertheless will often be confronted by clusters that have first been identified by alarmed residents of a neighborhood or employees of a particular building. Experience shows

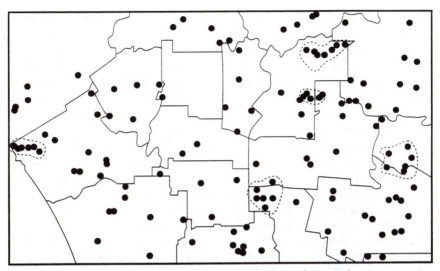

Five leukemia clusters constructed by selection of cases within tight boundaries are shown)

Figure 11.1   Childhood Leukemia Deaths, 1960–64, Central Los Angeles County,

that the vast majority of clusters reported by local citizens are examples of the Texas Sharpshooter at work.

The First Question: Is This Cluster Real?

A citizen reports a possible cluster to the County Health Department: is the cluster truly beyond the boundaries of chance? This is often a difficult question to answer, requiring sophisticated mathematical analysis (those with a technical interest might consult Wo93). Issues that must be addressed are the appropriate geographic and time boundaries that will be considered. Should we investigate the single street where a number of cases have been found, the entire neighborhood, or the community as a whole, and, how long a time period should we consider to be appropriate for the investigation of the suspect cluster?

An example of such an investigation was that conducted by the California State Department of Health Services (Ca91). In March 1984, a resident of the town of McFarland contacted the Kern County Health Department and requested an investigation of what appeared to be an unusual number of cancer cases among children within the preceding year in one part of the city. Six cases were identified. Subsequently, a house-to-house survey was conducted, searching for other cases. Adding cases that occurred in the following year, a total of 8 cases was found, whereas only 1.1 case would have been expected if rates in this population were the same as for the state as a whole. Such an excess would have occurred by chance alone only about two times in a hundred thousand. As a consequence, a survey was conducted among all 101 communities in the contiguous 4 counties. In that number of communities, one would expect roughly 5 communities to have rates greater than expected (even if they all had the same underlying rates). That was exactly the number found. One community would be expected to have rates outside the 99 percent confidence limits, and that was found— McFarland. Was McFarland just the statistical extreme that it appeared to be, or was there some cause operating in McFarland that caused these cases? The state thoroughly investigated the presence of contamination within the city, including EMF, and found no obvious chemical or physical cause for the cluster.

Raw numbers alone, such as those cited above in the McFarland case, may not be sufficient to determine the existence of a cluster— the epidemiologist will have to consider whether unusual risk factors may have contributed to this cluster. An example is the recent discovery of what appeared to be a cluster of breast cancer among women living on Long Island, New York. When factors known to increase risk for breast cancer were taken into account in estimating the expected number of cases of breast cancer, factors such as age at menarche, childbearing history, and prevalence of Jewish people (who are at increased risk), the observed number was no longer in excess (HHS92). The matter is still not entirely settled—the investigation is continuing.

The Second Question: What Caused This Cluster?

If a cluster is established as being a true cluster and is unlikely to have occurred by chance alone (chance always will remain a possibility), then one wishes to know whether there is a plausible explanation—what caused this? If the disease is infectious, the nature of the infection will suggest the source. Food-borne infections will suggest an investigation of local food supplies, of restaurants for example. If the disease is venereal, that would suggest another line of investigation. If the disease is cancer, as most often is the case with cluster reporting, one often searches for a physical or chemical agent in the environment. These investigations are generally fruitless. The primary reason is that known physical and chemical agents in the non-work environment rarely exist in concentrations high enough to cause cancer.

In fact, virtually all of the clusters reported to health officials either turn out not to exceed statistically expected numbers (i.e., they are not real clusters), or to be true clusters for which no cause can be ascertained.

Raymond Neutra, an epidemiologist who has reviewed the entire modern literature on investigations of neighborhood clusters, was able to find only a single case where an environmental (non-occupational) cause for a cancer cluster was found; this was in a village of 800 persons in rural Turkey where there was an unexpectedly high death rate from the rare cancer (mesothelioma) associated with exposure to asbestos-like materials (Ne90). In this remote geographic area there is an unusual outcropping of asbestos that is easily eroded by weathering, and the airborne dust produces high concentrations of asbestos in inhaled air.

Clusters Attributed to EMF

Several clusters of cancer have been attributed to EMF from power lines or utility facilities such as substations. Writing in a series of articles in the *NewYorker* magazine, Paul Brodeur reported several clusters of cancer and other diseases among populations alleged to be exposed to excessive EMF. One of these clusters occurred in a small town, Guilford, Connecticut, where Brodeur asserted that there was a cluster of disease among residents of Meadow Street near an electric utility substation. Such a facility will have measurable but not high levels of EMF around its periphery. The diseases Brodeur claimed to result from EMF exposure were a variety of different conditions as reported by the residents themselves. It would be surprising if one could not, on the basis of a door-to-door survey, find such a cluster of diseases in any neighborhood in the country. Is there a family anywhere that cannot report some disease in one or more members of the family, in persons who had previously lived in their house, or in neighboring houses? Thorough investigation by the

Connecticut State Health Department failed to confirm the cluster (Ba90a).

Brodeur also claimed to have identified clusters of cancer resulting from EMF at the Montecito and Slater schools in California (Br92c).

Montecito is a community in Santa Barbara County, California. In 1989, Montecito residents became concerned about an unusually high number of cases of leukemia among children aged 19 or younger. Analysis proved this number to be almost five times greater than expected during an eight-year period in a population the size of that of Montecito (Ca90). An extensive environmental assessment was conducted, including measurements of EMF in and around the elementary school. Those measurements revealed EMF levels to be similar to those in most schools and in most homes. Higher levels were found adjacent to the neighboring power line—similar to those near many power lines (Ca91)

The alleged cancer cluster at the Slater School in Fresno County, California, was not among students, but among teachers (there was no excess among children). The teaching staff strongly suspected these cases to be the result of EMF exposure from a neighboring power line. Twenty-eight cases of cancer were reported to the California Health Department among the 195 staff members who had been employed since the opening of the school in 1972. Upon investigation of these alleged twenty eight cases, only thirteen could be confirmed: in the remainder, the case could not be found, the person alleged to have cancer denied having cancer, or the person with cancer was diagnosed prior to employment at Slater.

Of the 13 confirmed cases, there was no consistent pattern of cancer site: breast (3), uterus (2), ovary (2), brain (1), melanoma (2), colon (2), and prostate (1), a mixture of cancer cases unlikely to result from a single cause.

The number of cases expected among the 195 staff members, if cancer rates were normal, would have been 6.9. Finding 13 cases, then, would be twice the expected number. A finding of twice the expected number of cases will occur in 25% of schools. Since California has 8,000 schools, it can be calculated that, on the basis of chance alone, 2,000 schools in California will have twice the number of expected cases (and 2,000 schools will have half the number of expected cases) (Ca93c).

Other Experiences With Childhood Cancer Clusters

In the 1960s, the finding that many animal cancers were of viral origin led to the suspicion that childhood cancer might also be of viral origin. The finding of cancer clusters among children, particularly of cases of leukemia, appeared to support the notion of an infectious etiology. A cluster of leukemia cases among children in Niles, Illinois, all of whom had attended the same high school, attracted national attention. Over subsequent years, a large number of clusters of childhood leukemia was investigated by the Centers for Disease Control. No cause for any of these clusters was found (Ca76), nor has any subsequently discovered cluster of childhood cancer been explained by association with local physical or chemical contamination. In the meanwhile, the evidence for a viral etiology of childhood cancer has faded, although the role of viruses in certain rare childhood cancers, particularly Burkitt's lymphoma, is now widely accepted.

Summary

While several clusters of cancer or other diseases have been suspected to be the result of exposure to EMF, none has been confirmed. In a few cases, the alleged cluster was statistically significant, but in no case was there found to be an association with EMF.

VI

EMF AND POSSIBLE HEALTH EFFECTS OTHER THAN CANCER

12

EMF and Reproduction

Harm to the developing fetus can result from a variety of insults: dietary deficiencies, exposure to certain chemicals (most commonly alcohol), viruses (e.g., German measles), or drugs (e.g., diethylstilbestrol, or DES). Many of these exposures may also affect the future reproductive capacity of either men or women.

CLASSIFYING REPRODUCTIVE EFFECTS

It is convenient to classify effects of environmental exposure according to the reproductive phase during which those effects appear:

- **Fertility.** Certain occupational exposures are known or suspected to adversely affect fertility (Ba93). Ionizing radiation at high doses will interfere with male fertility. An agricultural chemical, dibromochloropropane (DBCP), is also known to reduce male fertility, as are lead (in high concentrations), Kepone, and carbon

143

disulfide. Exposures to certain chemicals in the workplace, especially anesthetic agents, have been suspected of impairing female fertility (Ha91).

- **Damage to the fetus resulting in death (miscarriage or stillbirth) or in *malformations apparent at birth*.** Fertilization of the egg is followed by an extended period during which the newly formed organism begins rapid division and differentiation. Organ formation occurs in the human during the first third of intrauterine life. Toxic exposures during this period of organ formation can lead to death or malformations.

- Death of the early fetus is by no means rare. Between 15 and 35% of human conceptions result in death of the fetus and termination of the pregnancy (Br93). The causes of these early deaths are poorly understood, although many are thought to be the result of a defective fetus, i.e., one that is not viable, most often because of inherited genetic damage. The chance of such a miscarriage is related to the age of the parents, as reflected by the increasing difficulty of conception and completion of a normal pregnancy with advancing age of either the mother or the father. Factors related to miscarriage at later stages of pregnancy are parental age, history of previous miscarriage, chronic maternal disease (e.g., diabetes), maternal smoking or drinking, and stress.

- Malformations may result either from genetic factors (e.g., Down's Syndrome) or damage to the fetus itself. Many (almost 50) chemical and physical agents are known teratogens (agents capable of adversely affecting the development of the fetus). These include ionizing radiation, tobacco smoke, alcohol, and certain pharmaceuticals (e.g., thalidomide).Malformations visible at birth are not uncommon. Depending on the definition of a malformation, they may be found in as many as 7% of all births; about half are severe (Br93b).

- The precise effect of toxic exposures on the developing fetus will depend on several factors, including the stage of pregnancy at which the exposure occurs and the magnitude and duration of the exposure.

> • **Damage to the fetus resulting in effects that are not apparent at birth but** *appear during childhood.* Included are behavioral effects and cancer.
>
> The possibility that intrauterine exposures to the fetus can produce cancer in later life was first raised by the observation of vaginal cancer in women whose mothers were treated with the hormone DES during the pregnancy. There is now a growing body of literature that suggests, but by no means proves, that *pre-conception* exposures to either parent may produce cancer in the early life of the child (Sa90b).

In the discussions below, studies have been selected to illustrate the variety of studies of EMF and reproduction that have been reported. Comprehensive reviews of this literature are cited at the end of the chapter. References to the individual studies are cited in the reference list as a group; e.g., fertility studies are shown as (Fertility).

Each of the sections below begins with a review of the epidemiological studies, followed by a discussion of animal studies. Studies of human reproduction pose difficult issues such as the determination of reproductive practices, the identification of early pregnancy, and knowledge of the outcome of pregnancy. In the laboratory, animals can be bred at known times, and the outcomes of the pregnancies can be precisely determined. Therefore, animal studies of the effects of environmental agents on reproduction can be very helpful.

Fertility

In an early study, Wertheimer-Leeper attempted to determine the effect of EMF on the length of pregnancy, fetal loss, birth weight, and birth defects (We86). The study population was the 4,271 women who delivered in two different Denver hospitals in 1982. EMF exposure was estimated by a questionnaire inquiring about the use (during pregnancy) of an electric blanket or heated waterbed. Effects of EMF exposure on fetal growth and abortion rates were then estimated; fetal growth was impaired and abortion rates were increased among those with high exposure. These results have been questioned by others because of the abnormally low rate of defects among non-users, raising the question of bias in the selection of controls (Ch92). Furthermore, a study of EMF exposure during pregnancy among almost 3,000 women seen at Yale New Haven Hospital showed no effect on birth weight or intreuterine growth retardation (Br95).

In another study, Wertheimer and Leeper found that another source of EMF—household heating produced by electric ceiling coils—increased abortion and reduced fetal weight (We89a).

In a study of workers at electrical substations in Sweden, Bengt Knave and co-workers found that there were differences in family size and sex ratio (numbers of boys versus numbers of girls) among the offspring of the exposed men; however, these differences occurred before as well as after employment in substations (Kn79). The authors interpreted the study as negative, i.e., showing no relationship between work in electrical substations and sex ratio.

Video display terminals (VDTs) are now a common part of the business office—many workers spend their entire work day sitting in close proximity to these screens. The magnetic fields around these machines, which are like TV sets, are complex. The exposure to the operator from the 60-Hz signal may vary from 1 or 2 mG to as much as 10 mG, depending on the model of VDT and distance of the operator from the screen. (The fields decrease rapidly with distance, so that at a distance of several feet, the fields are insignificant, which is the reason that TV sets are not a matter of much concern).

At least a dozen studies of fetal loss among women VDT operators have been reported. The majority of these show no effects (these are referenced collectively as VDT, also Wi90b). In only one of these studies was exposure actually measured. These results led the author of one British study, also with no statistically significant findings, to conclude as follows: "In conclusion, women who work with VDTs are not at increased risk of clinically recognized spontaneous abortions. Given the consistency of our findings with those from recent studies it is reasonable to conclude that further research in this area is not warranted" (Ro92).

However, the most recent study of fetal loss among VDT operators, conducted in Finland, did find an association of occupational exposure to VDT's and fetal loss. Abortion rates among women who used different models of VDTs, with different exposure characteristics, were compared. This study showed no increase in spontaneous abortions for VDT users as a group, but when the women using VDTs with the highest exposures (greater than 9 mG) were examined separately, the abortion rate was statistically significantly increased compared with the lowest exposure group (less than 4 mG) (Li92).

This study suggests that the effect of high exposure may be obscured when studies examine all VDTs, without considering exposure levels associated with particular models.

The subject of EMF exposure and fertility in laboratory animals has been studied extensively. None of these studies found any effect on fertility (these references are grouped together in the reference section under Fertility).

Malformations

New York State maintains a registry of children born with congenital defects. Larry Dlugosz, then at the State University of New York, together with investigators from Yale and the Centers for Disease Control, utilized this registry to inquire of the mothers whether they had used electric blankets or electrically heated waterbeds during their pregnancies. The defects studied were cleft palate and certain defects of the brain and spinal cord. No effect of EMF on these conditions could be detected (Dl92).

While most studies of reproductive outcome are directed to effects on women, there are also a small number of studies of the offspring of men in electrical occupations. In a Swedish study, an increased number of malformations was found among the offspring of men employed in high-voltage switching facilities (No83). Numbers were small, however—there were 12 malformations among the 154 children of switchyard workers (8%), whereas, for example, there were 3 malformations among the children of 193 construction workers (2%). Various malformations were found, ranging from minor to major. Although there has been no subsequent study reported, a long-term prospective follow-up of Swedish utility workers is nearing completion.

Studies of malformations among children of VDT operators show a similar profile of results—the majority show no effects (Ku85, Er86a, Er86b, McD86a, McD88, Go88), while one does (Br90).

Studies designed to detect malformations in non human mammals exposed to either electric or magnetic fields showed no adverse effects on embryo development (references are grouped under Malformations). A variety of studies of electric and magnetic field exposures on the development of the chick embryo have been conducted, giving a variety of results (Ch92). However, because studies involving chicken eggs are so inconsistent, it is the judgment of most experienced scientists that the chicken egg is an unreliable model for predicting human effects from environmental exposures of any kind (Ch92).

Cancer Among Children of Parents Exposed to EMF

Two sets of studies have been conducted for the purpose of investigating possible effects of EMF exposure on cancer among offspring of the exposed: studies of children born to workers exposed to EMF prior to conception, and studies of children whose mothers were exposed to EMF during pregnancy.

Although it is difficult to conceive of a mechanism that might explain how occupational exposures to chemical or physical agents (such as EMF) among *men* prior to conception might produce cancer in the offspring following birth, a number of studies provide some evidence that such an effect may occur. Childhood brain cancer among offspring of EMF-exposed fathers has been examined. In several different case-control studies, an increase in childhood brain cancer among the children of fathers whose work presumably exposes them to EMF has been reported. Risk ratios are generally in the order of 2, but in certain subpopulations are considerably higher and sometimes reach statistical significance (Sp85, Wi88). Other studies have shown high but not statistically significant results (Jo89, Na88), or results have been negative (Bu90, Wi90b). As in most occupational studies, exposure assessment is based on job title, and therefore results of such studies must remain suspect.

There is only a single study that examines cancer in children specifically as a possible effect of EMF exposure to the in-utero child—the Denver study of David Savitz (Sa90c). The investigators reported an increased risk of both leukemia and brain cancer among children whose mothers used electric blankets during pregnancy.

Summary

Studies of possible effects of EMF exposure on each stage of reproduction (fertility, damage to the fetus apparent at birth, damage appearing after birth), both in human and animal studies, have been reviewed.

The EMF reproductive effects research literature has been reviewed by a number of investigators. Gary Shaw and Lisa Croen, both with the March of Dimes, conclude "Evidence is lacking for a strong association between a woman's use of a video display terminal (VDT) during pregnancy and spontaneous abortion. The evidence for a strong association between woman's use of a VDT and other adverse reproductive endpoints is also lacking, with some suggestive findings for congenital malformations and too few data to reach a conclusion about other measures of reproduction. With respect to low-level EMF exposure other than VDTs the paucity of data prevents one from determining whether there are reproductive health risks associated with such exposures" (Sh93a).

Robert Brent, a research pediatrician at the Jefferson Medical School, has thoroughly reviewed the EMF literature. He concludes (in part), "The population that has been most frequently studied are women exposed to VDTs, but their exposures are extremely low and frequently are at the level of the ambient EMF fields in a house or office. The results of epidemiological studies involving VDTs are generally negative for the reproductive effects that have been studied. Based on the number of studies, the exposure levels and the fairly consistent results, it can be argued that VDT epidemiological studies should no longer be given high priority (Br93b)."

Neil Chernoff and John Rogers of the Environmental Protection Agency, together with Robert Kavet of the Electric Power Research Institute, conclude, "Laboratory experimental and epidemiological results to date have not yielded conclusive data to support the contention that such fields induce adverse reproductive effects under the test or environmental conditions studied."

In spite of what appears to be a largely negative body of evidence, the matter of possible reproductive effects of EMF exposure cannot be considered closed, since many of the studies were conducted without adequate exposure assessment, and because our understanding of the biologically important parameters of magnetic field exposures remains weak; without such knowledge, design of definitive new studies will be difficult.

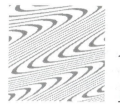

13

EMF and Neurobehavior

There are at least two good reasons for investigating the possibility of neurobehavioral effects of EMF. The first is the general observation that behavioral changes are often the most sensitive indicators of the harmful effects of exposure to an environmental agent. For example, extremes of heat, cold, and atmospheric pressure, and exposure to certain toxic agents, such as mercury and lead, all produce behavioral effects.

The second reason, more specific to EMF itself, is that function of the nervous system is strongly dependent on electrical signaling; that is, messages between the brain and other organ systems are sent by electrical signals through the conducting pathways of the nervous system. Is it possible that this signaling system could be influenced by field-induced currents?

IDENTIFYING NEUROBEHAVIORAL EFFECTS

If EMF (or any other environmental agent) does affect the nervous system, how might such effects be expressed? There are three main possibilities:

151

- Changes in the brain or other parts of the nervous system could occur, that is, structural changes visible either by eye or under the microscope.

- Neurological function might be altered, as reflected, for example, by changes in the secretion of melatonin from the pineal gland, or changes in the production of chemicals (neurotransmitters) that transmit signals across the gaps between nerve endings.

- Behavior of the organism could change. Altered ability to learn or discriminate is one example; symptoms of depression are another.

All of these examples of possible effects of EMF on neurobehavioral function have been subjected to some research, and many of these studies are mentioned elsewhere in this book. For example, effects of EMF on the pineal gland of the brain and its secretion of the hormone melatonin were discussed in Chapter 5, and possible effects of EMF on the behavior of electrical workers in Chapter 1.

This chapter begins with an examination of human studies, first epidemiological and then experimental (research involving human volunteers studied under laboratory conditions). These topics are followed by a review of animal studies.

Epidemiological Studies

The possibility of psychological effects of occupational exposure to EMF was raised early by Soviet scientists in the studies already referred to in Chapter 1. They found neurobiological effects among electrical workers exposed to high-intensity electric and magnetic fields. As a result of these reports, several Western psychologists and occupational physicians conducted both clinical and epidemiological studies of psychological functions among EMF-exposed populations, and they failed to confirm the Soviet findings (Ba86, Ga90).

That is where the matter remained until the publication by British investigators of a study reporting increased depression and suicide among persons living adjacent to transmission lines (Pe81). This was followed by studies, both of a population occupationally exposed to

EMF (Ba90b) and of a population exposed at home (McD86a), neither of which reported evidence of psychopathology.

Subsequently, a study of possible psychological effects of EMF was carried out by Charles Poole, an epidemiologist, and colleagues (Po93c). They investigated people who lived at the edge of a transmission-line **right-of-way**. Using telephone interviews, they assessed depressive symptoms as well as prevalence of headaches. They found that these symptoms were moderately associated with proximity to lines, the risk ratio for depression being 2.8 times greater for those living in proximity to transmission lines. The association could not be explained by socioeconomic variables.

The most recently published study, conducted in California, found no increase in depression among women living adjacent to a transmission line with high magnetic field exposures (mean = 4.86 mG), in comparison with women living one city block from the line whose exposure was 0.86 mG (McM94).

What we have, then, so typical of EMF research, is a collection of both positive and negative studies, with no consistent pattern of effects. There are three possible explanations for this inconsistency. The first is that there are no effects—that the studies showing effects are biased in some way. A second explanation is that the effects of EMF only occur under very specific circumstances (e.g., specific exposure conditions, interactions with other environmental agents) that existed in the studies in which effects were identified, but not in those where no effects were found. The last possibility is that individual human subjects vary considerably in their responsiveness to EMF. If the percentage of responsive persons in a population under study were small, then effects of EMF could be overwhelmed by the absence of effects in non-responsive individuals. These three possibilities are not mutually exclusive.

Laboratory Studies of Human Volunteers

One way of sorting out this issue is through the use of human volunteers studied in the laboratory under carefully controlled conditions.

The work of Charles Graham, a psychologist at the Midwest Research Institute; in Kansas City, Missouri, indicates that when human subjects are exposed in the laboratory to certain specific EMF exposure conditions (6–12 kV/m and 100 to 300 mG), their responses to stimuli are altered—they are slower, by fractions of a second, than those of unexposed volunteers. Whether this is of any clinical importance is not known, but if confirmed, it would support the possibility that the human nervous system is able to respond to environmental EMF (Gr90), even though many times greater than generally found in the environment.

Over the years, other investigators have examined complex behaviors of human subjects exposed to EMF. Studies of human behavior and alertness following exposure to magnetic fields for periods ranging to several days found no effects (Be73, Sa86). In another study, behavioral effects of magnetic field exposures were found, but these were transient and did not persist after exposure ended (Gi74).

Individual Variability?

There may be individuals who are sensitive to very low levels of EMF, i.e., lower than those to which most people respond. In Sweden, literally thousands of persons claim to be highly sensitive to very low levels of EMF. They cite burning sensations, faintness, palpitations, and rashes, among other symptoms, and indeed, because of the severity of these symptoms, some of them are unwilling to live in electrified communities. Study of these individuals has so far failed to explain their symptoms, but this research is continuing.

The notion of variation in individual responsiveness has some support from the laboratory. There are two studies, one of them not yet completed, that indicate considerable variation among human subjects in their ability to respond to and be influenced by EMF. One of these was a small study conducted some years ago by Barry Wilson at Battelle Northwest Laboratories, who examined changes in melatonin production in response to electric blanket use in human volunteers (Wi88) The other study, still in progress, is a study of melatonin response due to ambient magnetic fields in human volunteers, being conducted by Charles Graham. Neither study revealed any change in melatonin response due to EMF exposure for the study population as a whole. Both studies, however, appear to show effects in a subset of the individuals studied.

EMF and Circadian Rhythms

All animals, including human beings, undergo cyclical variations of biological functions throughout the 24-hour day.

This rhythmicity is referred to as a circadian rhythm. There is, of course, the obvious wake/sleep cycle, but in addition, many bodily functions vary from day to night. Pulse rate, blood pressure, and body temperature all decrease during sleep, as do some functions not so easily connected to bodily repose. For example, the response to drugs and X rays is altered during the night (we human beings are less sensitive to both while asleep).

If people are put into a cave or other environment in which the light is constant, the 24-hour rhythm slowly increases to about a 25-hour cycle. That is, without the cues of lightness and darkness, our biological clocks exhibit drift. However, even under constant illumination, human subjects can be kept on a 24-hour schedule through the appropriate scheduling of meals and other daily activities.

What controls biological rhythms? Where is the clock? Is there one clock or many? The best thinking today is that the clock is in a tiny portion of the brain, a switching station between the eyes and the pineal gland called the superoptic chiasm. It is apparently this clock that must be reset in adjusting to jet lag. There is some evidence that EMF can alter the synchronization of these rhythms. The evidence first surfaced some years ago with research in Germany conducted by Rutger Wever, a physicist working at the Max Planck Institute, in which volunteers spent some weeks in an underground bunker where light was carefully maintained and physiological functions were monitored. It was Wever who first observed that when humans are maintained without cues as to daily light cycles, they extend their cycles to an approximately 25-hour day (We92). He also found that relatively weak electric fields (2.5 V/m) could alter the synchronization of bodily functions, including secretion of melatonin, which is described elsewhere in this book.

Unfortunately, Wever's work with humans has never been repeated, although several scientists have examined the possibility that EMF exposure may alter circadian rhythms in non-human mammals. As so often is the case with research on laboratory animals, the results of these experiments are inconsistent and difficult to interpret. One reason, noted below, is that furry animals can sense electric fields, and may be responding to stress, i.e., any desynchronization noted could be the result of stress.

Behavioral Studies in Laboratory Animals

Study of the effects of electric and magnetic fields on the behavior of animals is complicated by the fact that furry animals used in laboratory studies can sense the electric component of the field at the intensities often used in experiments. This sensation is due to the induced oscillation of the hairs of the fur.

The evidence is that animals often avoid the electric field (although under certain circumstances, they seem to prefer it) (An90). It is therefore difficult if not impossible to determine whether electric-field induced changes in the behavior of these animals is the result of nonspecific stress of being in the field or the result of direct interaction with the nervous system. If the former is true, these studies have little value as predictors of behavior in nonfurry humans.

The majority of animal studies, whether of behavior, morphological changes, or neurotransmitter concentrations, have been conducted with high-intensity electric fields (greater than 5 kV/m) and with frequencies different from 60 Hz (These studies are extensively reviewed in Br92a). They may therefore not be that relevant to possible behavioral effects of electric or magnetic fields at levels normally encountered at power frequencies.

The response of laboratory animals to magnetic fields has not been as extensively studied as their response to electric fields. Results of the studies that do exist are mixed—some investigators find effects, others do not. The most recent study, carried out in the laboratory of Don Justesen at the Kansas City Veteran's Hospital in Kansas City, reports that behavioral conditioning of laboratory rodents can be influenced by exposures of 2 or more Gauss (Sm94).

In another study, rats were exposed to electric and magnetic fields for 20 hours per day of intrauterine life and 10 days of postnatal life. These animals showed lower response rates to stimuli both shortly after exposure and later in adult life. Whether this might be harmful or beneficial to these animals, or both, is not clear (Sa90a).

In still another study, pregnant rats were exposed to **pulsed** magnetic fields for 15 minutes, twice daily. The investigator found an alteration in behavior of the offspring (scent marking) at 120 days of age (McG90).

Summary

There are far fewer studies of EMF-related neurobehavioral effects than of studies related to cancer. Furthermore, there is great variation in the parameters of exposure used. There has been little replication of observed effects, when they were seen. At the moment, there is a consensus that few conclusions can be reached (Br92a).

VII
PUTTING IT ALL TOGETHER

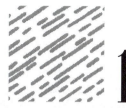

14

Quantifying the Risks of EMF: A Preliminary Effort

People often ask: "If the risk of EMF is real, how big a risk are we talking about?" People want to know, for example, whether EMF is as big a threat as cigarette smoking? In short, they want information that can help them put the risk into perspective.

In previous chapters reviewing the research on EMF health effects, the uncertainties in the data have been emphasized; in this chapter, for the purposes of conducting the exercise, the uncertainties will be ignored and the focus will be solely on the question of how big the risk *could* be if the risk were indeed real.

Measures of risk (relative risk, attributable risk) were previously described in Chapter 6. Risk refers here to the risk of specific diseases. The only disease for which quantitative estimates of increased risk from EMF exposure can be attempted is cancer. The following discussion focuses on cancer, first in children and then in adults.

EMF Cancer Risks—Children

First, let us look at what these measures of risk might be for children exposed to EMF, given our state of knowledge of those risks.

Risk Ratios. The estimated rate of cancer among children with high EMF exposures relative to the rate of those with low exposures is derived from studies using distance to power lines or "wire codes" as proxies or predictors of EMF exposure. Using either measure, the results of some studies described in Chapter 9 suggest that, if these studies are valid, high exposures could double the risk of childhood cancer. A doubling of risk would represent an increase in the risk of developing cancer (incidence) from 1 in 7000 to about 2 in 7000 per year. Risk of *death* from cancer for highly exposed children would rise from about 3 per 100,000 to about 6 per 100,000 per year.

Attributable Risk. Members of the New York Power Lines Project attempted to calculate the fraction of childhood cancer cases that may be attributable to EMF. They based their estimate entirely on the Savitz study. Using the formula for attributable risk shown previously, and extrapolating estimates of the risk and exposure information found in the Savitz study to the entire country, they calculated that 15% of all childhood cancer could be attributed to magnetic fields. This number is highly speculative because of the many assumptions involved, but is of value to public health officials in assessing the possible magnitude of the risks involved.

An estimated 8200 children were diagnosed with cancer in the United States in 1994 (Ca94). The number of cancer *deaths* was approximately 1600. Taking the attributable risk figure of 15% would suggest that about 1230 cases per year result from EMF exposure in the United States. Given the same assumptions, the annual number of cancer *deaths* among U.S. children attributable to EMF would be 240.

Anders Ahlbom made an estimate of the childhood leukemia that could be attributed to EMF from 220 and 400 kV transmission lines in Sweden (Ah92). He estimates that of the 70 cases that occur in Sweden each year, less than one case could be attributed to this source of magnetic field.

Both of these estimates, that for the United States cited in the previous paragraph and that for Sweden, should be considered to be highly uncertain.

Other Childhood Risks

Deaths among children are rare; of the some two million deaths per year in the United States, about twelve thousand occur among children. About 40 percent of these are due to accidents. Of the accidental deaths, 35 percent are due to motor vehicles, 23 percent are due to fires, 22 percent drowning, and the remainder are due to other causes. The second leading cause of death is heart disease; the third, cancer, accounts for about 12% of deaths among children.

Adult Cancer Risks

While there is little evidence of cancer in adults resulting from residential exposures to EMF, occupational exposure to EMF has been reported to contribute to mortality from several cancers (see Chapter 10). Leukemia and brain cancer are most prominent among these, but breast cancer and melanoma have also been reported.

Risk Ratios.   While estimates of relative risks of certain cancers among electrical occupations vary greatly from study to study, the risk ratios of cancer death averaged over these many studies are considerably less than twice that of non-exposed populations. For example, the two reviews cited in Chapter 10 (Savitz [Sa87] and Hutchison [Hu92]) both suggest a 20% increase in risk (a relative risk of 1.2).

Attributable Risk.   If we are to estimate the risk of cancer among electrical workers exposed to EMF, we must have some estimate of the numbers of workers exposed to varying levels of EMF in the workplace. While such information is still quite scanty, data from the Floderus study (Fl93) can be used for a "ballpark" calculation. As noted in Chapter 10, measurements of EMF were made for the large number of workers who were the subjects of the study. Results of that analysis suggest that half of the working population experience exposures above 2 mG, and that these persons have an increased risk of chronic lymphocytic leukemia.

Let us make a very conservative assumption although the only finding in the Swedish study was an increase in one kind of leukemia, for the sake of this calculation let us assume that these exposures are associated with an increase in risk of all leukemias and brain cancer as well, and that occupational exposures to EMF in Sweden are similar to those in the United States.

If, then, half of the workforce is exposed to levels of EMF that impose a small risk, and if that exposure were responsible for a 20% increase in all leukemias and brain cancer among members of the workforce, then the risk of these diseases attributable to EMF would be 10%, i.e., 10% of leukemia and brain cancer in the workforce may be the result of occupational exposure to EMF.

Leukemia occurs among U.S. adults at a rate of about 10 per 100,000 per year, whereas brain cancer occurs at about half that rate. If the U.S. workforce were taken to be 100 million, then the total numbers of cases (of leukemia and brain cancer) per year from all causes would be 15,000, and from the EMF exposure would be 1,500 cases (10%). This is quite likely an overstatement of the true impact, but no one has examined the matter carefully.

Some Risk Comparisons: Unlike the case with childhood cancer, where we know relatively little about environmental causes, there are many known causes of adult cancer. Some are shown in Tables 14.1 and 14.2. Table 14.1 shows some reported risk ratios, while Table 15.2 shows examples of some attributable risks.

It should be emphasized that there is a great deal of uncertainty in these numerical estimates. Both the magnitude of the risks assumed and the size of the populations exposed should be considered educated guesses.

Summary

Although the data is sparse, it may be of some use to attempt even a cursory assessment of the magnitude of risks that could be associated with exposures to EMF. Given our current state of knowledge, true risk estimates could be higher or lower, or, there could be no risk at all. Nevertheless, the most prudent judgment appears to be that risks of exposure, either to children or to electrical workers, are small compared to the already existing (baseline) incidence of cancer in the population.

Table 14.1 Risks for Cancers at Selected Sites in Association With Certain Exposures or Conditions

Cancer Site	Factor	High Risk	Low Risk	Risk Ratio
Stomach	Blood group	A	O	1.15
Nasopharynx	HLA system	BW46 antigen	Absence of BW46 antigen	1.8
Breast	Age at first birth	>30 years	<20 years	2.5
Breast	Ionizing radiation	>100 rads	No exposure	3.0
Pancreas	Cigarette smoking	>25 cigs/day	Nonsmokers	3.0
Bladder	Cigarette smoking	>25 cigs/day	Nonsmokers	5.0
Lung	Asbestos	Occupational exposure	No occupational exposure	5.0
Cervix	Cytological screening	Never screened	Negative result within three years	10
Esophagus	Alcohol consumption	>100 g ethanol/day, non smokers	<25 g ethanol/day, nonsmokers	17.5
		>100 g ethanol/day, 15-29 cigs/day	<25 g ethanol/day, nonsmokers	101.5
Lung	Cigarette smoking	>25 cigs/day	Nonsmokers	30
Liver	Hepatitis B virus	Carriers	Noncarriers	>100
Bladder	Benzidine and/or ß-naphthylamine	Occupational exposure	No occupational exposure	500
Leukemia	Melphalan	Ovarian cancer patients receiving >600 mg	No chemotherapy	20
Mesothelioma	Asbestos	Occupational exposure	No occupational exposure	>200

Table 14.2 Attributable Risks of Cancer Mortality From Exposures Considered by EPA

Type of Exposure	Estimated Annual U.S. Mortality
Depletion of stratospheric ozone	10,100
Indoor radon	5-15,000
Indoor pollutants (not radon)	500-7,000
Pesticides on food	3,000
Workplace EMF*	1,500
Toxic air pollutants	1,000
Inactive hazardous waste sites	500
Drinking water	240-591
Workplace chemicals	127
Consumer products	47-63
Total risk	22,197-44,153

*Not in original EPA list; see text

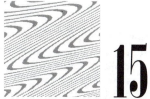

15

Reviews by
Government Agencies

For policy making and the guidance of future research, governments
and scientific organizations frequently assemble groups of scientists
to review an area of health-related research. Members of these review bodies are usually selected for their prominence as scientists
and for their freedom from any particular bias, rather than because
they have been actively engaged in this area of research. Several
such reviews of the EMF research have now been conducted; conclusions from those published since 1992 are excerpted below.

National Radiological Protection Board (NRPB92)

An Advisory Group on Non-Ionizing Radiation, chaired by Sir Richard Doll of the Imperial Cancer Research Fund Cancer Studies Unit
at Oxford University, concludes its review with the following:

"In summary, the epidemiological findings that have been reviewed
provide no firm evidence of a carcinogenic hazard from exposure of pa-

167

ternal gonads, the fetus, or adults to the extremely low frequency electromagnetic fields that might be associated with residence near major
sources of electricity supply, the use of electrical appliances, or work in
the electrical, electronic, and telecommunications industries. Much of
the evidence that has been cited is inconsistent, or derives from studies
that have been inadequately controlled, and some is likely to have been
distorted by bias against the reporting or publishing of negative results. The only finding that is at all notable is the consistency with
which the least weak evidence relates to a small risk of brain tumors.
This consistency is, however, less impressive than might appear, as
brain cancers in childhood and adult life are different in origin, arising
from different types of cell.

"In the absence of any unambiguous experimental evidence to suggest that exposure to these electromagnetic fields is likely to be carcinogenic, in the broadest sense of the term, the findings to date can be
regarded only as sufficient to justify formulating a hypothesis for testing by further investigation."

Doll has been quoted elsewhere as saying, "It doesn't look to be a
likely cause of cancer but you cannot put your hand on your heart
and say 'no biological effects,' so you cannot rule it out." (NS92)

In a supplementary statement published on June 9, 1994, contain-
ing comments on the most recent laboratory and epidemiological
studies, the Advisory Committee to the NRPB reiterated its earlier
position: "Thus, there is no persuasive biological evidence that ELF
electromagnetic fields can influence any of the accepted stages in
carcinogenesis. There is no clear basis from which to derive a meaningful assessment of risk, nor is there any indication of how any putative risk might vary with exposure" (NRPB94).

Expert Group on Non-Ionizing Radiation:
The Danish Ministry of Health (Da93)

This committee relied upon the British (NRPB92) report cited above
for all literature prior to the publication of the Swedish and the Danish studies of childhood cancer. The Committee's conclusion, in full,
is as follows:

"The opinion of the group is that both the Danish and the Swedish
study support the hypothesis of previous studies that children living
near high-current plants have an increased frequency of cancer, but the

results do not exclude the possibility that the association might be due to chance. If the increased cancer risk is due to 50-Hz magnetic fields, the uncertainty in the evaluation of exposures to magnetic fields would indicate too weak a correlation and thus result in a possible underestimation of potential risk.

"The expert group believed that neither the earlier nor the latest studies offer sufficient documentation to characterize 50-Hz magnetic fields in homes adjacent to high-current electricity supply plants as a cancer factor among children. The studies do not, however, allow this possibility to be dismissed.

"The group, therefore, finds no scientific reason for establishing standards with respect to high-current plants. New research results must be followed closely in the future."

Health Council of the Netherlands (Ne92)

"The Committee thinks that the results of the epidemiological studies as are now available do not justify the conclusion that there exists a relation between prolonged domestic or professional exposure to ELF EMF and adverse health effects. Present knowledge concerning the biological effects of ELF EMF furthermore does not clearly indicate the existence of such a relation. In other words, the Committee thinks that any evidence from currently available research is insufficient to support the hypothesis that exposure to ELF EMF generated by the electricity distribution system and by electrical household appliances and industrial equipment has any influence on the initiation or growth of malignancies, or on the course of pregnancy or fetal development."

Federal Committee on Interagency Radiation
Research and Policy Coordination (ORAU92)

This agency is chartered through the Federal Coordinating Council for Science in the Executive Office of the President of the United States. Its report was prepared by a committee of scientists coordinated by the Oak Ridge Associated Universities. The report, published in June of 1992, concludes with the following:

"This review indicates that there is no convincing evidence in the published literature to support the contention that exposures to extremely low-frequency electric and magnetic fields (ELF–EMF) generated by sources such as household appliances, video display terminals, and local power lines are demonstrable health hazards. Epidemiologic findings of an association between electric and magnetic fields and childhood leukemia or other childhood or adult cancers are inconsistent and inconclusive. No plausible biological mechanism is presented that would explain causality. Neither is there conclusive evidence that these fields initiate cancer, promote cancer, or influence tumor progression. Likewise, there is no convincing evidence to support suggestions that electric and magnetic fields result in birth defects or other reproductive problems. Furthermore, any neurobehavioral effects are likely to be temporary and do not appear to have health consequences."

French Academy of Medicine (Ro93)

In its report of a review of the health effects from EMF exposure, The Academy concluded that these represent "a very weak risk to the individual and do not represent a public health priority."

"The reported associations between EMF and certain pathologies like leukemias and other childhood and adult cancers cannot be supported by current epidemiologic data. However, to a certain extent, these associations remain plausible for childhood leukemia even in the absence of a known mechanism."

The Academy report also stated, "There is no conclusive evidence linking EMF to reproductive and teratogenic effects, or that EMF has a role in the initiation, promotion or progression of certain cancers, even though some data cannot exclude such a possibility."

Summary

The consensus of these reviews appears to be a general skepticism regarding the relationship of EMF to human health effects, particularly cancer. While the scientific method does not allow them to conclude that there is no harm from exposure to EMF, these scientific bodies are saying that evidence of harm from EMF exposure does not meet scientific standards of causation.

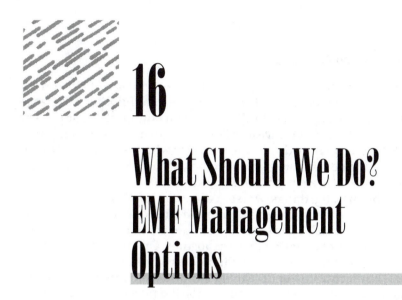

16

What Should We Do? EMF Management Options

Although the scientific committees cited in the last chapter have not advocated restricting exposures to EMF, the question of options for managing magnetic field exposures nevertheless deserves some consideration. Given the current state of knowledge, is there anything we can or should do, either as individuals or as communities? If evidence of harm from EMF exposure should become convincing, what might we do? What then are the options?

Granger Morgan of Carnegie Mellon University makes the practical observation that we have three options to respond to the still-uncertain evidence of harm from EMF:

- Do nothing at all.

- Undertake modest steps, i.e., those with relatively little cost, until the evidence of harm—or its absence—becomes clear.

- Undertake major national action to mitigate exposures.

Option 1: Do Nothing

Advocates of doing nothing argue that the evidence of harm from EMF is too fragmentary to do anything meaningful. Given the large number of real and unmet health needs that now exist, the argument continues, it would be a waste of resources to undertake mitigation of EMF, given that we do not know exactly what parameters of exposure need to be mitigated, and that the risk appears to be small, if it exists at all. It is even possible, in our state of ignorance, that we might be making things worse. Advocates of this point of view would say we really know little about the major contributors to exposure, which characteristics of exposure are harmful, or the most effective ways of lowering those exposures. Only now, for example, are we beginning to undertake the studies of major sources of exposure. The Electric Power Research Institute has completed a study of 1000 randomly selected U.S. homes for the purpose of identifying the major sources of exposure within those homes (EPRI93c). Until we know more about sources of exposure, the nature of sources that may produce harm, and the most cost-effective means of reducing risk, advocates of this option will say that it is difficult, if not impossible, to design a rational risk management program.

Option 2: The Middle Course

Granger Morgan has given a name to this middle course—"prudent avoidance." By prudent, he means taking simple steps that cost relatively little. By avoidance, he means reducing or avoiding EMF exposures. Even if the evidence of harm is weak, he asks, why not do these things, since they involve simple, but conscious choices to minimize risks?

Option 3: A Major Program

The third option on Granger Morgan's list, taking major national action, assumes that the risk is already adequately established for public policy purposes. Proponents of this option would urge that a major national program be undertaken quickly, even at great expense. This option has relatively few (but sometimes very vocal) supporters, and none who have specified exactly what programs of mitigation they would support, or at what cost.

One of the difficulties in implementation of this three-tiered system is that we do not have adequate definitions of *prudent* or of *reasonable costs*, nor is it clear just what the goals of a management program should be. For example, are we interested in reducing *fields* or reducing *exposure to people? The* strategy for reaching each of these goals could be very different. Transmission lines, for example, may be large sources of fields, but small sources of exposure to people since not many people live near transmission lines. Certain appliances (e.g., VDTs) or certain household wiring configurations (e.g., **knob and tube** wiring of the kind that is found in most older homes) may be relatively small sources of fields, but large sources of exposure since many people are exposed to these.

In undertaking a program of prudent avoidance, individuals and their families may want to consider both strategies—reducing fields in or near the home as well as reducing personal exposure by reducing time in the fields.

Options for Electric Utilities

Utilities may undertake reduction in fields to which the public is exposed, and may be able to reduce exposures to their employees by changes in work practices.

Some prudent avoidance options that have been suggested for new transmission lines are:

- Avoiding heavily populated areas

- Avoiding parks, schools, and other public facilities

- Using existing rights-of-way

- Limiting public use of rights-of-way

- Using line configurations that minimize exposures

- Undergrounding transmission lines

- Limiting power loading

The costs of each of these options will vary enormously from site to site (undergrounding is hardly an inexpensive option), and their effects on exposure to EMF often are not known with accuracy. Keith Florig of Resources for the Future, a Washington D.C. research institute, has provided some rough estimates of costs and the consequent

Table 16.1   Crude Estimates of the Costs and Cost–Effectiveness of Selected
Measures to Reduce EMF Exposures

Option	Total Cost (present value)	Cost per Exposure Avoided ($ per person)
Underground transmission lines near homes with transmission fields >1 mG	$200 billion	$ 75,000 per person
Buy out the 1 million homes with transmission line fields > 1 mG	$90 billion	$35,000 per person
Reduce average exposure from all existing transmission and distribution to <2 mG	$250 billion	$20,000 per person
10 mG limit on edge-of-right-of-way for all new transmission lines	$1 billion	$10,000 per person
Exposure "tax" on new transmission lines assessed for exposures >1 mG	$500 million	$2000 per person
Modify grounding system in homes where ground currents dominate exposure	$3-9 billion	$200-600 per person

exposure reduction, based on data derived from a survey of residential exposures conducted by Luciano Zaffanella (EPRI93c). The estimates are shown in Table 16.1. For each option shown, two values are calculated—the total cost and the cost per exposure avoided.

The first option shown in the table is undergrounding of transmission lines that produce an indoor exposure greater than 1 mG in nearby homes. The cost would be $200 billion, and the measure would affect 2.7 million persons. Although reductions in exposure would occur for all persons living in such homes, not all would have a reduction below 1 mG, since other sources of exposure might exist in these homes.

The estimated cost per person whose exposure is reduced by undergrounding, according to Florig, would be $75,000. The question of who would pay this cost is, of course, a dicey policy issue. Should the costs be spread among all clients of the utility, among those who may directly benefit, or among those in the community in which the transmission line undergrounding is done? If the individuals in these homes were to themselves pay these costs, under some circumstances their utility bills would become prohibitive.

For distribution lines, reconfiguring lines has relatively little effect on magnetic field levels. Research is focusing on better means of balancing the currents associated with the various phases (EPRI93b).

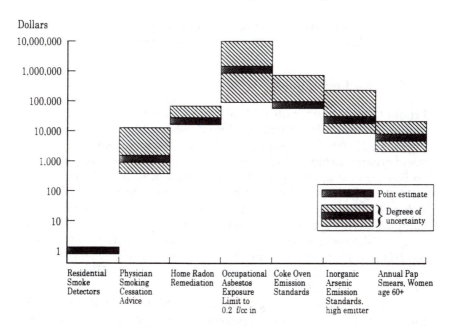

Figure 16.I   Comparison of Program Costs per Life Year Saved (1991 U.S.)
(Source: Harvard Center for Risk Analysis)

The question of how much we should spend to reduce the risks of
EMF exposure, or any other real or possible hazard, needs to be made
in conjunction with other expenditures for reducing risks. Examples
of other such costs are in Figure 16.1, which shows estimates of the
dollar costs per life saved by other prevention programs. Comparisons of this kind are useful in answering questions about reasonable
costs for hazard reduction.

Florig points out that given the money that we spend to reduce
other comparable risks, the most we could justify in reducing EMF
exposures, on the basis of other comparable risk reduction expenditures, would be $10 billion per year, an amount Florig estimates
would raise utility bills by 6%. How much magnetic field reduction
would that buy us? That would depend upon the choices we make
from the options shown in Table 16.1 (or other options).

In addition to the economic costs of exposure reduction, there may
be possible unforeseen risks associated with the mitigation itself. For
example, bringing electrical conductors closer together on towers, a

measure that would reduce magnetic field exposures, may pose added risks to linemen who must work around those lines.

Options for Individuals

Prudent avoidance for individuals might include alterations in behavior. An example is turning off your electric blanket after warming the bed but before getting into it. Other such options are to sit or stand greater distances from appliances, to reduce use of appliances, and to turn off appliances when they are not in use. Some newer models of electric blankets and computers have been redesigned to reduce EMF exposures. Digital clocks produce almost no exposure compared with the generally older electric clocks driven by small motors. Magnetic fields will vary considerably among appliance models. For example, at a distance of 10 inches from a microwave oven, the magnetic field may vary from a very few mG to over one hundred mG (EPRI93a).

In one survey, 64% of high magnetic field levels (greater than 3 mG) in homes resulted from household wiring, and the majority of these were the result of wiring errors (Wh93a). Working with a licensed electrician, the homeowner may be able to reduce magnetic field levels by eliminating improper grounding and by remedying improper electrical wiring. Research is now being conducted to search for superior means of grounding that may reduce fields as well as maintain safety; however, since grounding practices are prescribed by the National Electrical Code, any changes in grounding practices will have to first be approved by that organization.

More information about exposures from electrical appliances can be found in the EPA document, *EMF in Your Environment: Magnetic Field Measurements of Everyday Electrical Devices*. This publication (402–R–92–008) can be obtained free of charge by calling (202) 260–7751. Another source of information on reducing exposures in the home can be found in Wh93.

Options For Governments

The options discussed above, both for individuals as well as for utilities, are site specific and utilize technological fixes or changes in behavior. An option for government is to regulate exposures through the promulgation of guidelines or standards. Guidelines for electric

Table 16.2 Magnetic Field Limits At Power Frequencies

	Occupational	Public
Australia	As IRPA	As IRPA
Germany	50	50
UK - NRPB	20	20
USA - ACGIH	10	
USSR	18	
IRPA	5	1

NRPB National Radiological Protection Board
IRPA International Radiation Protection Association
ACGIH American Conference of Governmental Industrial Hygienists

and magnetic fields in the general environment have been pre-scribed in some countries, and these are shown in Table 16.2. Notice that different exposure levels are prescribed for workers and the general public. Occupational exposures are set higher, on the basis of an 8-hour day, rather than the 24-hour-per-day exposure limit for the general public.

Many jurisdictions have followed the guidelines established by the International Radiation Protection Association (IRPA), an inde-pendent scientific body that works closely with the World Health Association. The IRPA guideline for electric fields of 10 mA per square meter is based on the observation that such current densities occur naturally from biological functions (such as muscle move-ment). IRPA guidelines then translate these into specific magnetic field limits, as shown in Table 16.2 (Du92).

IRPA has been succeeded by the International Commission on Non-ionizing Radiation Protection. This agency reviewed the IRPA standards as recently as May 1993, and found no reason to alter the earlier standards.

Exposure guidelines for magnetic fields are far less common than those for electric fields, probably because substantial interest in magnetic fields as a possible health concern has only recently ap-peared. Another reason may be that while detectable effects of elec-tric field exposure (such as electric shock) are known to occur, there are no established harmful effects of magnetic fields at any level of exposure. Nevertheless, IRPA-recommended standards are 1000 mG for the public and 5000 mG for workers. The basis for these stan-dards is the levels of the body's own natural level of current density.

Two states (Florida and New York) have guidelines for magnetic fields around overhead power lines. The permissible levels in these states are between 150 and 200 mG at the edge of the rights-of-way. These levels are *not* based on evidence of harm at those levels, but are based on the magnitude of levels that now exist.

Having said all of this, it can be expected that individuals will reach a wide range of conclusions regarding the scientific issues as well as personal management options. Just as there is a wide range of responses to other potential health concerns, ranging from do nothing to extensive protective actions (rearranging bedrooms, rewiring, or even consideration of selling their house in favor of a lower exposure house). These are, of course, individual decisions, based on risk aversiveness, affluence, and interpretation of the risk data. It was a purpose of this book that people have available to them information with which to make these personal decisions in a way that seems most rational to each of them.

More Research

Regardless of views on policy, and while there is controversy about how much should be spent on research, most scientists agree that more research is desirable; however, they also agree that the quality of research must improve if the question of risk is to be resolved. The leading questions that need resolution are as follows:

- Is there a risk to human health from EMF exposure? What are these risks—for cancer (what kinds of cancer?), reproductive effects, neurobehavioral effects? Better epidemiological studies, particularly those with better means of exposure assessment, as well as control for confounding factors, are needed to answer this key question.

- Who is exposed? We still know very little about the important sources producing exposure to the population, both occupational and non-occupational, or the magnitudes of such exposures. Such information is being accumulated.

- What are the effects of EMF on cancer promotion in laboratory animals? Research of this nature has begun in many countries, but while many short-term tests have been completed, no cancer studies of animals exposed throughout their lifetimes have yet been completed.

- How does it work? What are the exposure parameters that are of importance biologically? If there is a problem, we need to know the conditions under which it exists. This requires some understanding of the mechanism, or at least reproducible effects in animals that are relevant to human health.

John Bailar, an epidemiologist at McGill University in Montreal, believes that until we get some of these basic questions resolved, we will continue to flounder. "We have seen the promulgation of a large number of hypotheses, of varying specificity and with widely varying support from data, about the effects of electromagnetic fields on health. Unfortunately it seems that none of these hypotheses have as yet been conclusively established or conclusively refuted. This has a further nonscientific but serious effect of leaving the whole field of study in some disrepute—few good scientists want to wade into a morass where nothing is ever settled" (Ba89). Bailar also suggests that it is time to begin thinking about "stopping rules" for ending EMF research. His point is that we may someday decide that this area of research has reached a dead end and that further research is unlikely to resolve uncertainty regarding the existence of risk from EMF exposure.

Currently, about $35 million per year is being spent worldwide on research, the majority of which is being carried out in the United States. The largest single sponsor of research in the United States is the Electric Power Research Institute (about $15 million per year). The largest federal agency research program is under the direction of the Department of Energy (which allocates about $5 million per year).

In 1992, Congress authorized a 5-year, $65-million program, to be funded equally by the federal government and by industry (Public Law 102–486). The program is to be under the direction of the Department of Energy and the National Institute of Environmental Health Sciences. A small portion of this money is earmarked for public education and policy research.

The question of how much research on EMF is justified is a difficult one, and one of some controversy. We have no adequate criteria with which to guide our allocation of research dollars to various public health needs. Some of the criteria that might be applied follow.

- How large a population is exposed? More properly, what is the distribution of exposures among members of the population?

- How convincing is the evidence of harm that does exist?

- How likely is it that a greater research effort will produce useful information?

- Are there researchers who are competent and interested in conducting research in this area?

- Is this an area of great concern to the public, who, in the final analysis, pay the costs of the research?

While most observers feel that an expanded EMF research program is justified, there is not universal agreement on the point. The recent Oak Ridge study participants argued that this area of research does not warrant an expanded research effort—the evidence does not justify it. They feel that, given the weakness of the evidence as it now exists, the level of research support (as described above) is about right.

What Can You Do? Keep Informed

Subscribe to a newsletter. Newsletters variously provide information on recent research, relevant meetings, government actions, and litigation. A variety are available:

EMF Health and Safety Digest, P.O. Box 14501, University Station, Minneapolis, MN 55414–0501

EMF Health Report,; c/o Information Ventures, Inc. 1500 Locust Street, Suite 3216, Philadelphia, PA 19102–4321

Microwave News, P.O. Box 1799, Grand Central Station, New York, NY 10163. (In spite of the name, this newsletter is largely devoted to power frequency news.)

Attend technical meetings. For the more technically minded, the Bioelectromagnetics Society (BEMS) sponsors an annual meeting each June and also publishes the journal, *Bioelectromagnetics*. Contact the Bioelectromagnetics Society, 120 West Church Street, Frederick, MD 21701; (301) 663–4252.

Each year, the Department of Energy, the Electric Power Research Institute; and others, sponsor an annual "EMF Contractor's Review," which is open to the public. Most of the scientists working in this field present short papers summarizing the status of their research. For information, consult one of the newsletters noted above. (Note: Most of these presentations are highly technical—they are not intended for a lay audience.)

Identify other sources of information.   Most but not all state health agencies have a radiation health office where you should be able to find technical expertise and answers to your questions. Your electric utility may be able to answer questions or provide written materials. The EPA provides information. Contact the U.S. Environmental Protection Agency, Public Information Center, 401 M Street SW, Washington, DC 20460; (202) 260–7751.

A recent EPA publication, *Questions and Answers About Electric and Magnetic Fields,,* is available (EPA document 402–R–92–009).

What Else Can You Do? Make Your Own Measurements

If you are concerned, find out what the magnetic field levels are in your home. Some electric utilities will make measurements for you. It is also possible that your state or local health department will make measurements for you. There are also private companies that will, for a price, make measurements. (There is no licensing process for such companies; caveat emptor!) For those who wish to follow this option, it must be emphasized that, while you will be able to compare readings in your home to those of others, these readings will otherwise be difficult to interpret. Are these readings high? Do they warrant any effort to reduce exposure levels? What will it cost to lower these levels, and what is the best way to do that? No one as yet has good answers to these questions.

One possibility is to obtain an instrument of your own. Several are available; you can get a list of them from the Edison Electric Institute, 701 Pennsylvania Avenue, Washington, DC 20004–2696; (202) 508–5000.

A very helpful guide for making measurements is available from Carnegie Mellon University. The guide is in two parts. *Part 1: Measuring Power Frequency Fields* and *Part 2: What Can We Conclude From Measurements of Power-Frequency Fields?* Copies can be obtained from Department of Engineering and Public Policy, Carnegie Mellon University, Pittsburgh, PA 15213.

Glossary

AC. The abbreviation for alternating current. An ac current, or an ac field, changes strength and direction in a rhythmically repeating cycle (in the United States, 60 cycles per second).

Ambient Magnetic Field. The background magnetic field level existing in the environment (such as in a home), without contribution from specific magnetic field sources such as appliances.

Ascertainment. (with respect to exposure assessment) The process of determining exposure, past and present, to the suspect agent, in this case, EMF. Also used to describe the process of determining the extent of the health efects produced by exposure.

Association. A relationship, generally demonstrated by statistical tests, between an exposure and a health effect. It does not necessarily imply cause and effect.

Attributable Risk. The percentage of cases of disease or death that can be attributed to a particular cause. For example, 22.8% of deaths among children aged 1–4 are attributed to fires.

Bias. Any trend in the collection, analysis, interpretation, or publication of a study that can lead to conclusions that are different from the truth. Unlike the common use of the word, the existence of bias in a study does not imply a psychological prejudice.

Carcinogen. A chemical, biological, or physical agent capable of producing cancer.

Case-Control Study. An investigation of the extent to which a group of persons with a specific disease (the cases) and comparable persons who do not have the disease (the controls) differ with respect to exposures to putative risk factors.

Charge. The electrical property of matter that is responsible for creating electric fields. Charge may be positive or negative. Electric fields begin on positive charges and end on negative charges. Similar charges repel each other. Dissimilar charges attract each other.

Circadian Rhythms. Biological processes or functions (such as blood pressure or temperature) that rise and fall throughout the day, generally rising during the day and falling during the night. Some functions, such as the secretion of certain hormones, rise at night.

Conductor. A material that allows the free flow of electricity, such as the wires on transmission lines. Metals are particularly good conductors.

Cohort Study. A cohort is a group of people who have something in common. For example, they may be people who were born in the same year or people who work in the same factory or live in the same neighborhood. A cohort study, then, is the study of health or disease in such a cohort where the exposures of individuals to a suspect agent are known.

Confidence Interval. A range of values for a variable of interest, such as a rate, constructed so that this range has a specified probability of including the true value of the variable. The specified probability is called the confidence level, and the end points of the confidence interval are called the confidence limits. For example, an odds ratio of 3.0 may have *confidence limits* of 2.0–4.0 with 95% *confidence level*, and is commonly written as 3.0 (2.0–4.0).

Confounding. A situation in which an observed association between an exposure and a disease is influenced by variables other than those under study. A confounding factor will be correlated with both the exposure and the health outcome.

Contact Current. The current that flows in the body when a person touches a conducting object (e.g., wire fence or a refrigerator) that has a voltage induced in it because it is in an ac field or because of leaking insulation.

Current. The flow of electrically charged particles. The unit is the ampere (A).

Distribution Line. A power line used to distribute power in a local region. Distribution lines typically operate at voltages between 5 and 35 kV—much lower than the voltages found on transmission lines. However, the currents found on some distribution lines can be comparable to transmission line currents.

Dose. In respect to EMF, refers to the specific characteristics of exposure which are effective in producing biologic alterations, whether harmful or not.

Ecological Study. An ecological study is one in which groups, rather than individuals, are compared. In general, results of such studies have less validity than studies in which individuals are compared.

Electric Field. The region in which a force exists between two objects or particles *because* they are charged. An electric field is present around any source where an electric potential difference, or voltage, exists. Electric current need not flow for an electric field to exist. For example, when an appliance is plugged into an outlet, a voltage exists across the cord and device, and an electric field is created even though the appliance may not be operating.

Electric Field Strength. The force on a stationary unit positive charge at a point in an electric field: the magnitude of an electric field vector. The unit is volts per meter, V/m.

Electrical Workers. Persons employed in several occupations that have been assumed on the basis of the job title to have a high probability of exposure to EMF. Examples are electricians, welders, and electronics technicians.

Epidemiology. The study of the occurrence and distribution of disease in populations for the purpose of understanding the causes of disease.

Exposure. The joint occurrence in space and time of a person and an agent (such as EMF).

Exposure Assessment.   An activity to define the magnitude, frequency, duration, route, and extent of exposure of an individual or a population to an agent in the environment.

Exposure-Response Assessment.   The process of estimating the relation between the exposure of a substance and the risk of an adverse health effect.

Field.   A physical quantity that takes on different values at different points in space. Examples are gravitational fields and magnetic fields.

Frequency.   The number of complete cycles of a periodic waveform per unit time. The units of frequency are hertz (Hz), equivalent to cycles per second.

Gauss.   A unit of magnetic flux density. A milligauss (mG) is one thousandth of a Gauss.

Grounding.   Connecting a charged conductor to something that will accept excess charge, such as the earth or a water pipe.

Ground Current.   An electrical current that flows through the ground (or on pipes) rather than on wires.

Harmonics.   Multiples of the fundamental frequency used for a particular power source. 60-Hz harmonics are 120 Hz, 180 Hz, 240 Hz, etc.

Hertz (Hz).   The unit for frequency. The number of complete cycles of a waveform per second (cycles per second).

Incidence.   A measure of new cases of disease appearing in a certain time frame, usually a year. Incidence is expressed as a rate.

Initiating Agent.   A chemical or physical agent capable of initiating cancer in cells. The mechanism of initiation is thought to be the production of permanent damage to the genetic material of the cell.

Intermittency.   In the context of this book, intermittency refers to interrupted as opposed to constant fields.

Job Title: A commonly used surrogate for exposure to an environemntal agent in epidemiological studies is the study of persons in a particular job. For example, a study examining the possible health effects of EMF might examine health among electricians.

Knob and Tube Wiring.   An older form of household wiring in which the two conductors are separated, thus producing higher magnetic fields than with the more-modern wiring systems in which the two conductors are wound together in the same sheath.

kV. Abbreviation for kilovolt; a thousand volts.

Leukemia. A disease characterized by an excess of white blood cells in the blood-forming organs and in the circulating blood. May be of the acute form, which can be rapidly fatal, or of the chronic form, which can be a prolonged and relatively benign disease.

Lymphocytic Leukemia. A kind of leukemia marked by an excess of lymphocytes, a type of white cell in the blood.

Magnetic Field. A vector quantity that describes the forces of interaction between electric currents and includes contributions of both macroscopic and microscopic currents.

Model. A condition or disease occurring in laboratory animals, similar to one occurring in humans, that is useful in testing theories or causes of disease.

Mutagenesis. A change in the characteristics of an organism produced by an alteration in the hereditary material. The alteration may involve a change in one or more chromosomes, ranging from a deletion or rearrangement, or the alteration may be a minute rearrangement in a single gene – a gene mutation.

Myelogenous Leukemia. A type of leukemia marked by an excess of myelocytes, a type of white cell in the blood.

Nanovolts. One millionth of a volt, or, one thousandth of a millivolt.

Negative Study. A study in which the risk found among the exposed population is not statistically different from that of the unexposed population. Accordingly, a positive study is one in which a significant difference in disease outcome is found among the exposed population.

Odds Ratio. The exposure odds ratio is the ratio of the odds in favor of exposure among the cases to the odds in favor of exposure among the controls. Within each group, the odds is the ratio of the numbers of exposed and non-exposed individuals.

Parts Per Million. When the entire sample, or population, is divided into a million parts, the number of those parts that are of a specified nature. For example, if it is said that drinking water contains chlorine in a concentration of ten parts per million, it is meant that every million gallons contains ten gallons of chlorine.

Power Frequency.   The frequency at which electrical power is generated. In North American,the frequency is 60 cycles per second. In Japan and Europe, the frequency is 50 cycles per second.

Progression.   A stage in cancer evolution following the stage of promotion. It is in this latter stage that the cancer enters the final stage of malignancy.

Promotion.   The second hypothesized stage in the development of cancer. The conversion of initiated cells into tumor cells. Examples of promotional agents are estrogens, high-fat diet, alcohol, and certain mineral oils.

Publication Bias.   A form of bias whereby study results are differentially reported depending on the direction and strength of the findings. For example, it appears to be more likely that positive studies (those reporting an effect of exposure or therapy) will be reported than will negative studies (those in which no significant findings are reported). This bias results in the perception of a greater strength of association than in fact would exist if all studies were published.

Pulsed Magnetic Field.   In contrast to the smooth sinusoidal field found with electric power, a pulsed field repeatedly rises abruptly to a high level and then abruptly falls to the previous level.

Relative Risk.   The *ratio* of the risk in an exposed population with that in a similar but unexposed population.

Reproductive Effects.   Toxic effects on reproduction, which may include, but not be limited to, alterations in sexual behavior, onset of puberty, fertility, gestation, parturition, lactation, pregnancy outcomes, or delayed effects in the newborn resulting from exposures to the mother or father.

Resonance.   The transfer of energy (e.g., sound, wind, light) from one system to another system having similar frequency characteristics. A simple example —the vibration of a violin string will initiate vibration in a string of a second nearby violin.

Right-of-Way.   The strip of land on which a transmission line is built. In some countries high-voltage transmission lines pass directly over buildings, but in the United States buildings are not allowed on the rights-of-way of high-voltage lines. The width of the right-of-way varies with line voltage and from state to state. Some power companies own the land; some do not.

Risk.   The probability that a person will experience an adverse effect from some activity or exposure.

Risk Assessment.   The use of available information to evaluate and estimate exposure to a substance and its consequent adverse health effects.

Risk Factor.   An aspect of personal behavior or lifestyle, an environmental exposure, or a genetic characteristic that is known from epidemiological data to be associated with adverse health effects.

Risk Management.   Policies undertaken to mitigate risk, based on information regarding benefits and risks of exposure to certain substances or agents.

Risk Ratio.   The ratio of the probability of a risk in some designated population, in comparison with the probability of that risk in another population. An odds ratio is a particular kind of risk ratio. For example, if the *risk ratio* for lung cancer among cigarette smokers is increased in comparison with nonsmokers, then the risk ratio will be elevated.

Sinusoidal.   A waveform having periodic oscillations in the shape of a sine wave.

Spot Measurement.   A magnetic field measurement taken at discrete points in space and time. Spot measurements do not provide any information about the spatial or temporal variation of a magnetic field, which will vary as the load or current varies.

Statistical Significance.   A finding of an epidemiological study is considered to be of statistical significance if, according to certain assumptions and based on mathematical probability, the finding has a low likelihood of being due to chance.

Substation.   Utility facility at which voltage is transformed, generally from higher to lower voltage.

Surrogate.   A substitute. An exposure surrogate is defined as a factor, other than a direct measure, that is assumed or has been shown to be representative of exposure to an agent.

Teratology.   The scientific study of the causes of congenital malformations—birth defects.

Time-Varying Fields.   Electric and magnetic fields that vary over time (as distinguished from the earth's constant or static field, which does not vary).

Time-Weighted-Average: The average exposure over a given period of observation.

Transformer.   Devices used to change or transform the voltage on electric power lines either up or down. Transformers may be seen as cylinders on power poles. Much larger transformers are seen in electrical substations.

Transmission Line.   The high-voltage portion of the utility system that transports power at high voltages. When the power is to be distributed, its voltage is reduced to lower distribution voltages.

Transient.   An abrupt increase in the electrical or the magnetic field. Usually the result of switching on motors or other appliances.

Tumor.   Any abnormal growth. Need not be cancerous. Tumors are often harmless, but can be harmful if they interfere with normal function, as in a brain tumor, or may become harmful if they become cancerous.

Voltage.   The electrical potential energy difference per unit charge between two points. The unit is called the volt (V). A volt is defined as the potential difference between two points in a circuit when a current of one ampere flows through the circuit and the power dissipated in the circuit is one watt.

Wire Code.   An exposure surrogate that uses physical parameters of nearby electric power facilities to rank presumed background residential magnetic field levels.

References

Ab92   Abelson P, Remediation Of Hazardous Waste Sites, Editorial, Science, 1992;255:901

Ad91   Adair R, Constraints On Biological Effects Of Weak Extremely-Low-Frequency Electromagnetic Fields. Physical Reviews 1991;43:1039–1048

Ah92   Ahlbom A, Journal of the Swedish Medical Association (in Swedish) 1992;89:4371–4374

Ah93a   Ahlbom A, And Feychting M, Studies Of Electromagnetic Fields And Cancer: How Inconsistent? Environmental Science And Technology 1993; 27:1018–1020

Ah93b   Ahlbom A, Feychting M, Koskenvuo M, Olsen JH, Pukkala E, Schulgen G And Verskasal P, Pooling Three Nordic Studies On EMF And Childhood Cancer (Letter) Lancet 1993

Am90   Ames B, And Gold L, Too Many Rodent Carcinogens: Mitogenesis Increases Mutagenesis. Science 1990;249:970–1

Am93   American Council On Science And Health. Holiday Dinner Menu. 1993 Broadway, New York, Ny 10023–5860

AMA93   American Medical Association, Council on Scientific Affairs, Diet and Cancer: Where Do Matters Stand? Archives of Internal Medicine 1993;153:50–56

191

An90   Anderson LE, Interaction of ELF Electric and Magnetic Fields with
        Neural and Neuroendocrine Systems. In Wilson B, Stevens, R, And
        Anderson L, (Eds.) Extremely Low Frequency Electromagnetic
        Fields: The Question Of Cancer. Battelle, Richland, WA 1990 pp
        139–157

APS95   American Physical Society. Power Line Fields and Public Health.
        529 14th St. NW, Washington, DC 20045

As92   A Celebration Of Isaac Asimov: A Man For The Universe. Skeptical
        Inquirer 1992;17:30–48

Ba86   Baroncelli P, Battisti S, Checucci A, Comba P, et. al., A Health Ex-
        amination Of Railway High Voltage Substation Workers Exposed
        To ELF Fields. American Journal Of Industrial Medicine
        10;45–55:1986

Ba89   Bailar JC, Research On The Health Effects Of Electromagnetic
        Fields: Science, Uncertainty And Stopping Rules. Proceedings Of
        The American Statistical Association Conference On Radiation And
        Heatlh VIII, Held At Copper Moutain, Colorado, July 9–13, 1989.

Ba90a   Banks RS, Cluster Analyses Do Not Support Calamity on Meadow
        Street Claims. Robert S. Banks Associates. EPRI EN–7067. October
        1990.

Ba90b   Baris D, Armstrong, B, Suicide Among Electric Utility Workers In
        England And Wales. British J. Ind Med 1990; 47:788–78

Ba92   Basset AL, Bioelectromagnetics In Service Of Medicine. Bioelectro-
        magnetics 1992;13:7–17

Ba93   Baranski B, Effects Of The Workplace On Fertility And Related Re-
        productive Outcomes. Environmental Health Perspectives.
        Suppl.101 (Suppl 2):81–90, (1993)

Be73   Beisher DE, Grissett JD And Mitchell RE, Exposure Of Man To Mag-
        netic Fields At Extremely Low Frequency. NAMRL–1180. Pensaco-
        la, Fl. Naval Aerospace Medical Research Laboratory. 1973

Be91   Beniashvili DS, Bilanshavili VG And Menabde MZ, Low-Frequency
        Electromagnetic Radiation Enhances The Induction Of Rat Mam-
        mary Tumors By Nitrosomethyl Urea. Cancer Letters 1991;61:75–9

Be94   Bennett WR, Jr. Cancer and Power Lines.Physics Today April, 1994.
        pp 23–29

Bl90a   Blackman C ELF Effects on Calcium Homeostasis. In, Wilson B., Ste-
        vens R., And Anderson L. (Eds.) Extremely Low Frequency Electro-
        magnetic Fields: The Question Of Cancer. Batelle, Richland, 1990
        pp187–210

Bl90b   Blask D, The Emerging Role Of The Pineal Gland And Melatonin In
        Oncogenesis. In, Wilson B., Stevens R., And Anderson L. (Eds.) Ex-
        tremely Low Frequency Electromagnetic Fields: The Question Of
        Cancer. Batelle, Richland, 1990

Br 85   Broadbent DE, Broadbent MHP, Male J and Jones MRL, Health of Workers Exposed to Electric Fields. British Journal of Industrial Medicine. 1985; 42: 75–84

Br89   Brodeur P, Currents Of Death: Power Lines, Computer Terminals And The Attempt To Cover Up Their Threat To Your Health. Simon And Schuster, New York, 1989

Br 90   Brandt LPA and Nielsen CV, Congentital Malformations Among Children of Women Using Video Display Termianls. Scandinavian Journal of Work, Environment and Health. 1990;16:329

Br92a   Brady JY, And Reiter RJ, Neurobehavioral Effects. In, Health Effects Of Low-Frequency Electric And Magnetic Fields. Prepared By An Oak Ridge Associated Universities Panel; For The Committee On Interagency Radiation Research And Policy Coordination. Oak Ridge Associated Universities. Oak Ridge TN, 1992, pp VII–1–56

Br92b   Brainard GC, Project Review Of Electric And Magnetic Fields And Melatonin. Review Of A Symposium, July 8–9, 1992, jointly sponsored by The Electric Power Research Institute And The United States Department Of Energy

Br92d   Brodeur P, The Cancer At Slater School. The New Yorker, December 7, 1992, pp. 86-119

Br93a   Bracken TD, Kheifets LI And Sussman SS, Exposure Assessment For Power Frequency Electric And Magnetic Fields (EMF) And Its Application To Epidemiologic Studies. Journal Of Exposure Analysis And Environmental Epidemiology 1993;3:1–22.

Br93b   Brent RL, Gordon WE, Bennett WR and Beckman DA, Reproductive And Teratologic Effects Of Electromagnetic Fields. Reproductive Toxicology 1993;7:535–80

Br93c   Brodeur P, The Great Power-Line Cover-Up. Boston, Little, Brown And Company. 1993

Br95   Bracken MB, Belanger K, Hellenbrand K, et al., Exposure to Electromagnetic Fields During Pregnancy With Emphasis on Electrically Heated Beds. Association With Birthweight and Intrauterine Growth Retardation. Epidemiology 1995; 6:263–170

Bu90   Bunin G., Ward E., Kramer S., et. al., Neuroblastoma And Parental Occupation. American Journal of Epidemiology1990; 131:776–780

Ca62   Carson RL, Silent Spring. Houghton-Mifflin, Boston, 1962

Ca76   Caldwell GG and Heath CW Jr., Case Clustering in Cancer Southern Medical Journal 1976; 69: 1580–1602

Ca90   Investigation of the Montecito Leukemia and Lymphoma Cluster. Final Report, February 1990, and Supplementary Report May 1991. California Department of Health Services. Environmental Epidemiology anfd Toxicology Program.

Ca91   The Four County Study of Childhood Cancer Incidence: Interim Report #2. California Department of Health Services. Environmental Epidemiology and Toxicology Program. October 21, 1991.

Ca93a   Cain CD, Thomas DL, and Adey WR, 60-Hz 60 Hz Magnetic Field
         Acts As Co-Promoter In Focus Formation Of C3h/10t1/2 Cells.
         Carcinogenesis 1993;14: pp. 955–60

Ca93b   Cain CD, Thomas DL, Jimenez L, et. al., Dependence Of 60-Hz Mag-
         netic Fields Strength On Copromotion Of Focus Formation. (Ab-
         stract). Bioelectromagnetics Society Fifteenth Annual Meeting, Los
         Angeles, CA June 13–17, 1993 P.75

Ca93c   California Department of Health Services.An Evaluation of an Al-
         leged Cancer Cluster Among Teachers at the Slater School Between
         1973 and 1992. Environmental Epidemiology and Toxicology Pro-
         gram. 1993

Ca94   Cancer Facts – 1994. American Cancer Society. 1599 Clifton Road,
         NE. Atlanta, GA 30329–4251

Ch81   Cheney M. Tesla: Man Out Of Time. Englewood Cliffs, N.J. Prentice-
         Hall, 1981

Ch92   Chernoff N, Rogers JM, Kavet R. A Review Of The Literature On Po-
         tential Reproductive And Developmental Toxicity Of Electric And
         Magnetic Fields. Toxicology 1992;74:91–126

Co83   Conti P, Gigante GE, Cifone MG et. al.,. Reduced Mitogenic Stimula-
         tion Of Human Lymphocytes By Extremely Low Frequency Electro-
         magnetic Fields. Febs Lett. 1983;162:156–160

Co89   Coleman MP, Bell CMJ, Taylor Hl, Primic-Zakelj M. Leukaemia And
         Residence Near Electricity Transmission Equipment: A Case- Con-
         trol Study. Br J Cancer 1989;60:793–798

Cr85   Crump K, Mechanisms Leading To Dose-Response Models. In,
         Principles Of Health Risk Assessment. Ricci P, Ed. Prentice Hall, pp.
         321–372, 1985

Da88   Davis MK, Savitz DA, and Graubard BI. Infant Feeding and Child-
         hood Cancer. The Lancet, Aug 13, 1998, pp365–368

Da93   Danish Ministry Of Health, Expert Group On Non-Ionizing Radi-
         ation. May 1993. English Summary

De90   Demers P., Thomas D., Rosenblatt K., et. al., Occupational Exposure
         To Electromagnetic Radiation And Breast Cancer In Males. Ameri-
         can J. Epidemiol 1990; 132: 775–776

Dl92   Dlugosz L, Vena J, Byers T, Sever L, Bracken M, And Marshall E.,
         Congenital Defects And Electric Bed Heating In New York State: A
         Register-Based Case-Control Study. American Journal Of Epide-
         miology 1992;135:1000–1011

Do81   Doll R, And Peto R. The Causes Of Cancer, Quantitative Estimates
         Of Avoidable Risks Of Cancer In The United States Today. Journal
         Of The National Cancer Institute, 1981;66:1192–1308

Do93   Dovan T, Kaune WT, And Savitz DA. Repeatability Of Measure-
         ments Of Residential Magnetic Fields And Wire Codes. Bioelectro-
         magnetics 1993;14:145–159

Du78   Dubrov AP, The Geomagnetic Field And Life, New York, Plenum
          Press, 1978
Du92   Duchene AS, Lakey JRA, And Repacholi MH (Eds.) IRPA Guide-
          lines On Protection Against Non-Ionizing Radiation. Hightown NJ
          Mcgraw Hill 1992
Ea91   Easterbrook PJ, Berlin JA, Gopalen R, And Matthews DR, Publica-
          tion Bias In Clinical Research. Lancet April 13, 1991 337;867–72
EEI94   Evaluating EMF. Quarterly Public Opinion Review. First Quarter,
          1994, Edison Electric Institute, Washington, DC
EPRI92   Electric Power Research Institute. Electric And Magnetic Field Ex-
          posure, Chemical Exposure, And Leukemia Risk In "Electrical Oc-
          cupations." EPRI TR–101723 Prepared By University Of Southern
          California. December 1992
EPRI93a   Electric Power Research Institute. EMF In American Homes. EPRI
          Journal April/May 1993 8 Pages
EPRI93b   Electric Power Research Institute. Managing Magnetic Fields. EPRI
          Journal July/August 1993. pp7–13
EPRI93c   Electric Power Research Institute. Survey Of Residential Magnetic
          Field Sources (2 Vols). EPRITR–102759–Vi, September 93
EPRI94   Electric Power Research Institute. Occupational EMF Exposure As-
          sessment. Environmental Division. Resource Paper. February, 1994
Er86a   Erickson A, and Kallen B, An Epidemiological Study of Work With
          Video Screens and Pregnancy Outcome. I. American Journal of In-
          diustrial Medicine 1986;9:447–475
Er86b   Erickson A, and Kallen B., An Epidemiological Study of work With
          Video Screens and Pregnancy Outcome. II American Journal of In-
          dustrial Medicine 1986;9:459–475
Ev77   Evans AS., Limitations Of Koch's Postulates. Lancet 1977; 2:1277
Fe88   Feinstein, A. Scientific Standards In Epidemiologic Studies Of The
          Menace Of Daily Life. Science, 1988;242:,1197–1203.
Fe92   Feychting M, Ahlbom A, Magnetic Fields And Cancer In People Re-
          siding Near Swedish High Voltage Power Lines. Stockholm, Swe-
          den: Karolinska Institute, Institute Of Environmental Medicine;
          1992 June
Fe93   Feychting M, Ahlbom A, Magnetic Fields And Cancer In Children
          Residing Near Swedish High-Voltage Power Lines. American Jour-
          nal Of Epidemiology 1993;138:467–81
Fe94   Feychting M, Ahlbom A. Magnetic Fields, Leukemia and Central
          Nervous System Tumors in Swedish Adults Residing Near High-
          Voltage Power Lines. Epidemiology 1994;5:501–509

Fertility Studies

          Conti R. 1989. Enel's Research Activity On Possible Biological Ef-
          fects Of 50 Hz Electromagnetic Fields. Results And Plans Of A

Large Research Program. Alta Frequenza Vol. 58: 395–402 (Specially Devoted To The Leghorn Chickens)

Fam, WZ, 1980. Long-Term Biological Effects Of A Very Intense 60 Hz Electric Field On Mice. Ieee Transactions On Biomedical Engineering, Vol. Bme–27: 376–381

Kowalczuk C.I. 1990. Dominant Lethal Studies In Male Mice After Exposure To A 50 Hz Electric Field. Bioelectromagnetics. 11: 129–138

Le Bars H., Laboratory Long Term Studies On Animals Subjected To An Electric 50 Hz Field. Ennergia Elettrica 1990; 17: 343–349

Marino A.A. et. al., The Effect Of Continuous Exposure To Low Frequency Electric Fields On Three Generations Of Mice. Experientia 1976;15: 565–566

Mikolajczyk H, Effect On TV Sets Electromagnetic Fields On Rats. Work With Display Units 1976;86. Elsevier: 122–128

Rommereim D.N., 1987. Reproduction And Development In Rats Chronologically Exposed To 60 Hz Electric Fields. Bioelectromagnetics 8: 243–258

Rommereim D.N., et. al., 1990. Reproduction, Growth, And Development Of Rats During Chronic Exposure To Multiple Field Strengths Of 60 Hz Electric Fields. Fundamental And Applied Toxicology. 14: 608–621

Seto Y.J. 1984. Investigation Of Fertility And In-Utero Effects In Rats Chronically Exposed To A High Intensity 60 Hz Electric Field. IEEE Transactions On Biomedical Engineering. Bme. 31: 693–701

Sikov M.R. (1987). Developmental Studies Of Hanford Miniature Swine Exposed To 60 Hz Electric Fields. Bioelectromagnetics 8: 229–242

Zusman I. (1990) Effects Of Pulsing Electromagnetic Fields On Prenatal And Postnatal Development In Mice And Rats: In Vivo And In-Vitro Studies. Teratology 42;157–170

Fl93   Floderus B, Persson T, Stenlund C, Wennberg A. Ost A, And Knave B. Occupational Exposure To Electromagnetic Fields In Relation To Leukemia And Brain Tumors. A Case-Control Study In Sweden. Cancer Causes And Control 1993;4:465–476

Fr90   Frazier ME, Reese JA, Morris JE et. al., Exposure Of Mammalian Cells To 60 Hz Magnetic Or Electric Fields: Analysis Of DNA Repair Of Induced Single Strand Breaks. Bioelectromagnetics 1990; 11:229–234

Fu80   Fulton J., Cobb S., Preble L., Leone L., Forman E., Electrical Wiring Configurations And Childhood Leukemia In Rhode Island. Am J Epidemiol. 1980;111(3):292–296

Fu93   Fumento M, Science Under Siege. New York, William Morrow, 1993

Ga90   Gamberale F. Physiological And Psychological Effects Of Exposure To Extremely Low-Frequency Electric And Magnetic Fields On Humans. Scand J Work Environ Health 1990;16(Suppl 1):51–4

Ge84   Geddes LA, A Short History Of The Electrical Stimulation Of Excitable Tissue Including Electrotherapeutic Applications. A Supplement To The Physiologist, 1984;27:S1–S47

Gi74   Gibson RS, and Moroney WF. The Effect of Extremely Low Frequency Radiation on Human performance: a Preliminary Study. NAMRL–1195. Pensacola FL Naval Aerospace Medical Research Laboratory 1974

Gl68   Glass AG, Hill JA, And Miller RW. Significance Of Leukemia Clusters. The Journal Of Pediatrics. 1968;73:101–107

Go88   Goldhaber MK, Polan MR and Hiatt RA. The Risk of Miscarriage and Birth Defects Among Women who Use Video Display Terminals During Pregnancy. American Journal of Industrial Medicine 1988;13:695–706

Go90   Gough M, How Much Cancer Can EPA Regulate Away? Risk Analysis 1990:10:1–6

Go91   Gould SJ, Bully For Brontosaurus; Reflections In Natural History. Chapter 12: The Chain Of Reason Versus The Chain Of Thumbs Pp. 183–197 New York, Norton, 1991

Go93a   Goldstein BD, Demak M, Northridge M, and Wartenberg. Risk To Groundlings Of Death Due To Airplane Accidents. Risk Analysis 1992;12:339–341

Go93b   Goodman, R. And Henderson, A. The Effect Of Electric And Magnetic Fields On Transcription In Cultured Human Cells. EPRI TR–102860 December 1993

Go93c   Gould JL, Birds Lost In The Red. Nature 1993;364:491–2

Gr85   Greenberg RS, And Schuster JL. Epidemiology Of Cancer In Children. Epidemiology Reviews. 1985;7:22–48

Gr90   Graham C. Immunological And Biochemical Effects Of 60-Hz Electric And Magnetic Fields In Humans, Final Report, 1990 Midwest Research Institute, 425 Volker Blvd. Kansas City, MO 64110–2299

Gr93   Graham C, Cook MR, Cohen DH Riffle DW, et. al., EMF Suppression In Human Volunteers. (Abstract) Contractors's Review, October 31–Nov 4, 1993 Savannah Georgia

Gu93   Guenel P, Raskmark P., Andersen JB, And Lynge E. Incidence Of Cancer In Persons With Occupational Exposure To Electromagnetic Fields In Denmark. British Journal Of Industrial Medicine 1993;50:758–764

Ha91   Hatch M, And Marcus M. Occupational Exposures And Reproduction. In Kiely M, (Ed) Reproductive And Perinatal Epidemiology. CRC Press. Boca Raton, 1991, Pp 131–143

Ha92   Hatch M. The Epidemiology Of Electric And Magnetic Field Exposures In The Power Frequency Range And Reproductive Outcomes. Paediatric And Perinatal Epidemiology 1992;6:198–214

He81   Henderson, B., Ross, R., And Pike, M. Toward The Primary Prevention Of Cancer. Science, 1981:254;1131–1138

He88   Herbst AL, The Effects In The Human Of Diethylstilbestrol (DES) Use During Pregnancy. In, Miller RW, Watanabe S, Fraumeni JF, et. al., (Eds.) Unusual Occurrences As Clues To Cancer Etiology. Japan Scientific Societies Press, Tokyo, Taylor And Francis, London, pp. 67–75, 1988

HHS92 Breast Cancer On Long Island, New York prepared For The New York State Department Of Health By The Centers For Disease Control And Prevention, December 17, 1992, U.S. Department Of Health And Human Services, Public Health Service.

Hi65   Hill AB, The Environment And Disease: Association Or Causation? Proc Royal Soc Med 1965;58:295–300

Hi95   Hitchcock RT, Patterson RN. Radio-Frequency and ELF Electromagnetic Energies. New York, Van Nostrand Reinhold 1995

Ho95   Horton WF, Goldberg S. Power Frequency Magnetic Fields and Public Health. Boca Raton, CRC Press 1995

Hu92   Hutchison G. Carcinogenic Effects Of Exposure To Electric And Magnetic Fields. In: Future Epidemiologic Studies Of Health Effects Of Electric And Magnetic Fields. Report No. EPRI TR–101175, Palo Alto, California, Electric Power Research Institute 1992 September,

Ja92   Jackson JD, Are The Stray 60-Hz Electromagnetic Fields Associated With The Distribution And Use Of Electric Power A Significant Cause Of Cancer? Proceedings Of The National Academy Of Sciences 1992;89:3508–3510

Ja93   Jansson E. Re: Congenital Defects And Electric Bed Heating In New York State: A Register-Based Case-Control Study. (Letter) American Journal Of Epidemiology 1993;137:585–587

Jo89   Johnson CC and Spitz M. Childhood Nervous System Tumors: An Assessment of Risk Associated With Paternal Occupations Involving Use, Repair, or Manufacture of Electrical and Electronic Equipment. International Journal of Epidemiology 1989;18:756–82

Jo93   Jones TL, Shih CH, Thurston DH, Ware BJ, and Cole P. Selection Bias From Differential Residential Mobility as an Explanation For Associations of Wire codes with Childhood Cancer. Journal of Clinical Epidemiology 1993;46:545–548

Ka82   Kalmijn AJ Electric And Magnetic Field Detection In Elasmobranch Fishes. Science 1982;218:916–918

Ka92   Kavet R, Silva JM, And Thornton D. Magnetic Field Exposure Assessment For Adult Residents Of Maine Who Live Near And Far Away From Overhead Transmission Lines. Bioelectromagnetics 1992; 13:35–55

Ka93   Kato M, Honma K, Shigemitsu T, And Shiga Y. Effects Of Exposure To A Circularly Polarized 50-Hz Magnetic Field On Plasma And Pineal Melatonin Levels In Rats. Bioelectromagnetics 1993;14:97–106

Ki85   Kirschvink J., Jones D., And Macfadden B. Magnetite Biomineralization And Magnetoreception In Organisms. New York, Plenum Press, 1985

Kl89   Kline J, Stein Z, And Susser. Conception To Birth: Epidemiology Of Prenatal Development. New York, Oxford University Press. 1989

Kn79   Knave B, Gamberale F, Bergsttrom S et al. Long Term Exposures to Electric Fields. A Cross Sectional Epidemiologic Investigation of Occupationally Exposed Workers in High-Volatge Substations. Scandinavian Journal of Work, Environment and Health. 1979;5:115–25

Kn88   Knudson AG. Rare Cancers: Clues To Genetic Mechanisms. In, RW Miller, et. al., (Eds) Unusual Occurrences As Clues To Cancer Etiology. Jan Science Society Press, Tokyo. 1988;221–231.

Ko72   Korobsova V, Morozov Y, Stolorov M, And Yacub Y. Influence Of The Electric Field In 500 And 750 KV Switchyards On Maintenance Staff And Means For Its Protection. Presented At The International Conference On High -Tension Electric Systems. August 28–Sept 6, 1972; Paris, France Paper 23–06

Ko93   Koppett L. Quoted In The San Francisco Chronicle, December 31, 1993

Kr94   Kraut A, Tate R, and Tran N. Residential Electric Consumption and Childhood Cancer in Canada (1971–1986) Archives of Internal Medicine. 1994;49:156–159.

Ku85   Kurpa K, Holmberg K, Pantela K, Nurminen T and Saxen L. Birth Defects and Exposure to Video Display Terminals During Pregnancy. Scandinavian Journal of Work, Environment and Health 1985;11:353–356

Le90   Lewis J. Employment In Electrical Occupations And The Risk Of Neurological Tumors. Doctoral Dissertation, University Of Texas School Of Public Health, 1990

Le91a   Leeper E, Wertheimer N, Savitz D, et. al., Modification Of The 1979 "Denver Wire Code" For Different Wire Or Plumbing Types. Biolectromagnetics 1991;12:315–318

Le91b   Lerchl A, Nonaka KO, And Reiter RJ. Pineal Gland "Magnetosensitivity" To Static Magnetic Fields Is A Consequence Of Induced Electric Currents (Eddy Currents). J. Pineal Research 1991;10:109–116

Le95   Leiss JK, and Savitz, D. Home Pesticide Use and Childhood Cancer: A Case-Control Study. American Journal of Public Health. 1995;85:2449–252

Li78   Lichtenstein S, Slovic P, Fischoff B, Layman M, And Coombs B. Judged Frequency Of Lethal Events. Journal Of Experimental Psychology: Human Learning And Memory 1978;4:551–578

Li80   Lilienfeld A, Lilienfeld D. Foundations Of Epidemiology (2nd Ed.) Oxford University Press New York, 1980

Li85   Lin RS, Dischinger PC, Conde J, And Farrell K. Occupational Exposures To Electromagnetic Fields And Brain Tumors. Journal Of Occupational Medicine 1985;27:413–419

Li89   Lin SR, Lu PY, An Epidemiologic Study Of Childhood Cancer In Relation To Residential Exposure To Electromagnetic Fields. Abstract From DOE/EPRI Contractors Meeting. Portland Oregon 1989

Li90   Liboff AR, The Ion Cyclotron Resonance: A Physical Basis For The ELF Interaction With Biological Systems. In, Wilson, B., Stevens, R., And Anderson, L. (Eds.) Extremely Low Frequency Electromagnetic Fields: The Question Of Cancer. Battelle, Richland, 1990

Li92   Lindbohm M, Hietanen M, Kyronen P, et al. Magnetic Fields of Video Display Terminals and spontaneous Abortion. American Journal of Epidemiology 1992;136:1041–51

Lo91   London S., Thomas D., Bowman J., Sobel E., And Peters J. Exposure To Residential Electric And Magnetic Fields And Risk Of Childhood Leukemia. Amer J Epidemiol 1991;134:923–37

Lo94   Loomis DP, Savitz DA, and Ananth CV. Breast Cancer Mortality Among Female Electrical Workers in the United States. Journal of the National Cancer Institute. 1994;86:921–925

Lu93   Lucier GW. Risk Assessment: Good Science For Good Decisions (Editorial) Journal Of The National Institute Of Environmental Health Sciences 1993;101:366

Ly88   Lyle DB, Ayotte RD, Sheppard AR, And Adey WR. Suppression Of T-Lymphocye Cytotoxicity Following Exposure To 60-Hz Sinusoidal Electric Fields. Bioelectromagnetics 1988;9:903–313

Malformations

Coulton LA, And Barker AT, The Effect Of Low Frequency Pulsed Magnetic Fields On Chick Embryonic Growth. Phys Med Biol 36: 369–381

Fam WZ,. Long-Term Biological Effects Of Very Intense 60 Hz Electric Field On Mice. IEEE Transactions On Biomedical Engineering,1980: Vol. Bme–27: 376–381

Knickerboker G.G. (1967). Exposure Of Mice To A Strong AC Electric Field: An Experimental Study. IEEE Transactions Power App. System Pas–86: 498–505

Stuchly M.A.. Teratological Assessment Of Exposure To Time Varying Magnetic Field. Teratology 38: 461–466

Ma91   Matanoski GM, Breysse PN, And Elliott EAF. Electromagnetic Field Exposure And Male Breast Cancer. (Letter) 1991;337:737

Ma92a Maddock BJ, Guidelines And Standards For Exposure To Electric And Magnetic Fields At Power Frequencies. 1992. Session Panel 2–05 Cigre 3 – 5 Rue De Metz 75010 Paris

Ma92b   Matanoski GM, Breysse PN, Elliott E, Obrahms GI, And Lynberg M. Leukemia In Telephone Linemen. Prepared For The Electric Power Research Institute, Final Report, Palo Alto, Ca.December 1992.

Ma93   Matanoski G, Elliott E, Breysse P, Lynberg M. Leukemia In Telephone Linemen. American Journal Of Epidemiology 1993;137 (6):609–19

McC93a   McCann J, Dietrich F, Rafferty C, Martin A, A Critical Review Of The Genotoxic Potential Of Electric And Magnetic Fields, Mutation Research, 1993;297:61–95

McD86a   McDonald AD Cherry NM Delorme C, McDonald JC Visual Display Units and Pregancy: Evidence From the Montreal Survey. Journal Of Occupational Medicine 1986;28:1226–1231

McD86b   McDowall ME, Mortality Of Persons Resident In The Vicinity Of Electricity Transmission Facilities. British Journal Of Cancer 1986;53:271–279

McD88   McDonald AD, McDoanld JC Armstrong B, et al Work With Visual Display Units in Pregancy. British Journal of Industrial Medecine 1988;13(6):695–706

McG90   McGivern RF Sokol RZ, Adey R. Prenatal Exposure To A Low- Frequency Electromagnetic Field Demasculinizes Adult Scent Marking Behavior And Increases Accessory Organ Weights In Rats. Teratology. 1990;41:1–8

McL92   McLeod KJ, And Rubin CT, The Effect Of Low-Frequency Electrical Fields On Osteogenesis. Journal Of Bone And Joint Surgery, 1992;74–A:920–929

McL93   McLean JRN, Thansandote DW, Lecuyer DW, et. al.,. The Effect Of Magnetic Fields On Tumor Co-Promotion In Sencar Mouse Skin. Abstract P–B–60. Bioelectromagnetics Society Fifteenth Annual Meeting, Los Angeles, CA June 13–17, 1993 P.153

McM94   McMahan S, Ericson J, And Meyer J. Depressive Symptomatology In Women And Residential Proximity To High-Voltage Transmission Lines. American Journal Of Epidemiology 1994;139:58–63

Me93   Mevissen M, Stamm A, Butenkotter S, et. al.,. Effects Of Magnetic Fields On Mammary Tumor Development Induced By 7,12– Dimethylbenz (A)Anthracene In Rats. Bioelectromagnmetics 1993;14: 131–143

Mi85   Milham S, Mortality In Workers Exposed To Electromagnetic Fields. Environmental Health Perspectives. 1985;62:297–300

Mi92   Milunsky A, Elcickas M,, Willett W, Jick SS, And Jick H. Maternal Heat Exposure And Neural Tube Defects. Journal Of The American Medical Association 1992;268:882–885

Mi93   Miller BA, Ries LAG, Hankey BF, Kosary CL And Edwards BK. Cancer Statistics Review; 1973–89. National Cancer Institute. NIH Pub. No.92–2789, 1993

Mo83   Morris JE, And Phillips RD. Effects Of 60-Hz Electric Fields On Specific Humoral And Cellular Components Of The Immune System Bioelelctromagntics 1983;4:294

Mo92a   Modan B, Wagener DK, Feldman JJ et.al. Increased Mortality From Brain Tumors: A Combined Outcome Of Diagnostic Technology And Change Of Attitude Toward The Elderly. Am Journal Of Epidemiology 1992;135:1349–57

Mo92b   Morgan MG, Prudent Avoidance. Public Utilities Fortnightly March 15, 1992, pp. 26–29

Mo92c   Mouchawar GA, Bourland JD Nyenhuis JA, Geddes LA, Foster KS, Jones JT And Graber GP. Closed-Chest Cardia Stimulation With A Pulsed Magnetic Field. Med.& Biol. Eng. & Comput. 1992;30:162–8

Mu93   Murphy J, Kaden DA, Warren J And Sivak A. Power Frequency Electric And Magnetic Fields: A Review Of Genetic Toxicology. Mutation Research 1993;296:221–240

My85   Myers A., Cartwright R., Bonnell J., Male J., And Cartwright S. Overhead Power Lines And Childhood Cancer. Technical Report, Proceedings Of The International Conference On Electric And Magnetic Fields In Medicine And Biology. London: The Institute Of Electrical Engineers; 1985. Pp. 126–130

Na88   Nasca P., Baptiste M., Maccubbin P. et.al. An Epidemiologic Case-Control Study Of Central Nervous System Tumors In Children And Parental Occupational Exposures, Am J Epidemiol 1988; 128:1256–1265

NAS83   Risk Assessment In The Federal Government: Managing The Process. Committee On The Institutional Means For Assessment Of Risks To Public Health. Washington, Dc, National Academy Press, 1983

NAS93   Committee On Risk Assessment Methodology. Issues In Risk Assessment National Academy Press, Washington, DC, 1993

Ne90   Neutra, R. Counterpoint From A Cluster Buster Am Journ Epi, 132, pp. 1–8, 1990

Ne92   Health Council of the Netherlands.Extremely Low Frequency Electric and Magnetic Fields and Health. The Hague, April 8, 1992

NIH93   Cancer Statistics Review 1973–1989. Miller BA, Ries LAG Hankey BF, Kosary CF, And Edwards BK(Eds) US Department Of Health And Human Services, Public Health Service, NIH, NCI Bethesda, Md 20892–9903. NIH Publication No. 92–2789

No83   Nordstrom S., Birke E., Crustavson L. Reproductive Hazards Among Workers In High Voltage Switch Yards. Bioelectromagnetics 1983; 4:91–101

NRPB92 Electromagnetic Fields And The Risk Of Cancer. Report Of An Advisory Group On Non-Ionizing Radiation. National Radiological Protection Board Chilton, Didcot, Oxon Ox11orq, England 1992

NRPB94 Electromagnetic Fields And The Risk Of Cancer. Supplementary Report Of An Advisory Group On Non-Ionizing Radiation National Radiological Protection Board. Chilton, Didcot, Oxon Ox11orq, England, 12 April, 1994

NS92　New Scientist, 21 November, 1992, pg. 35

NYT93　Brody J, Personal Health. New York Times, February 24, 1993.

O'C88　O'Connor ME, And Lovely RH (Eds.), Electromagnetic Fields And Neurobehavioral Function. New York, Alan R. Liss Inc. 1988

OR92　Health Effects Of Low-Frequency Electric And Magnetic Fields. Prepared By An Oak Ridge Associated Universities Panel For The Committee On Interagency Radiation Research And Policy Coordination. ORAU 92/F8, June 1992. Oak Ridge Associated Universities, Oak Ridge TN

Ol90　Olcese JM, The Neurobiology Of Magnetic Field Detection In Rodents Progress In Neurobiology 1990;35:325–330

Ol93　Olsen JH, Nielsen A, And Schulgen G. Residence Near High- Voltage Facilities And The Risk Of Cancer In Children. British Medical Journal 1993;307:891–895

OR93　ORAU Panel On Health Of Low Frequency Electric And Magnetic Fields. Letter To The Editor, Science 1993;260:13–14

Pa92　Parker JE, And Winters W. Expression Of Gene-Specific RNA In Cultured Cells Exposed To Rotating 60-Hz Magnetic Fields Biochem, Cell Biol. 1992;70:237–241

Pe81　Perry F., Reichmanis M., Marino A., Becker R. Environmental Power-Frequency Magnetic Fields And Suicide Health Physics 1981;41:267–277

Pe93　Petridou E, Kassimos D, Kalmanti M, Kosmidis H, Haidas S, Flytzani V, Tong D, And Trichopoulis D. Age Of Exposure To Infections And Risk Of Childhood Leukemia. British Medical Journal 1993;307:774

Pe94a　Penrose JF. Inventing Electrocution. Invention and Technology Spring 1994. pp. 35–44

Pe94b　Peters J, Preston-Martin S, London S, et al. Processed Meats and Risk of Childhood Leukemia. Cancer Causes and Control 1994:5: 195–202

Pe95　Pearson R, Wachtel H, And Ebi K. Childhood Cancer Risk in Relation to Residential Environment and Life Style Factors that Are Associated With Wire Codes. (Abstract) Presented at Bioelectromagnetic Society Meeting, June 18–22, 1995. Boston, MA p. 87

Pi93　Pitot HC. The Dynamics Of Carcinogenesis: Implications For Human Risk. CIIT Activities 1993;13:1–6 Chemical Industry Institute Of Toxicology, Research Triangle Park, NC

Po92　Pollack H, From Microbes To Microwaves: Autobiography Of A Medical Man. San Francisco Press, San Francisco, 1992

Po93a   Pokorny G, EMF The Process Of Dialogue. Electric Perspectives 1993; May–June:68–80

Po93b   Polk C, Application Of Electric And Magnetic Fields In Bone And Soft Tissue Repair. In, The Electrical Engineering Handbook Dorf RC, (Ed) CRC Press, Boca Raton 1993 Pp 2329–2341

Po93c   Poole C, Kavet R, Funch DP et.al. Depressive Symptoms And Headaches In Relation To Proximity Of Residence To An Alternating Current Transmission Line Right-Of-Way. American Journal Of Epidemiology 1993;137:318–30

Pr93   Preston-Martin S, Peters JM, Yu MC, Garabrant DH, And Bowman JD. Myelogenous Leukemia And Electric Blanket Use. Bioelectromagnetics 1993;9:207–213

Pr94   Preston-Martin S, Navide W, Thomas D, Bowman J, And Sobel E. Epidemiological Study of Brain Tumor in Children and Exposure to Magnetic Fields: Los Angeles County, 1989–1994. Final Progress Report, November 7, 1994 Department of Health Services Contract # 89–97575/819669 1989–94

Ra93   Rannug A, Holmberg B, Ekstrom T, Hannson Mild K. Rat Liver Foci Study On Coexposure With 50 Hz Magnetic Fields And Known Carcinogens. Bioelectromagnetics 1993;14:17–27

Re79   Reichmanis M., Perry F., Marino A., Becker R. Relation Between Suicide And The Electromagnetic Field Of Overhead Power Lines. Physiol Chem And Physics 1979; 11:395–403

Re92   Reilly JP, Electrical Stimulation And Electropathology. Cambridge University Press, New York, 1992

Re93   Rensberger B, Forget Horoscopes! Consult Old Sunspots. International Hearld Tribune, May 27, 1993, p.8

Ri79   Rish WR And Morgan G. Regulating Possible Health Effects From AC Transmission Line Electromagnetic Fields. Proc IEEE1979; 67:1416–1427

Ro84   Rowbottom M, And Susskind C. Electricity And Medicine: History Of Their Interaction. San Francisco Press, San Francisco Ca 1984

Ro88   Ron E, Modan B, Boice JD, et.al. Tumors Of The Brain And Nervous System After Radiotherapy In Childhood. New England Journal Of Medicine. 1988:319:1033

Ro90a   Rommereim DN, Rommereim RL, Sikov ML, Buschbom RL, Reproduction, Growth, And Development Of Rats During Chronic Exposure To Multiple Field Strengths Of 60 Hz Electric Fields. Fundamental And Applied Toxicology. 1990;14: 608–621

Ro91a   Rosenfeld SS, And Massey EW. Epidemiology Of Primary Brain Tumor. In, Anderson DW (Ed). Neuroepidemiology: A Tribute To Bruce Schoenberg. Boca Raton, CRC Press, 1991 pp.121–144

Ro91b   Ross DJ. EMF and Public Policy: Balancing Interests Of Customers, Shareholders, And The Public. Electricity Journal 1991;4#3:46–53

Ro92   Roman E, Beral V, Pelerin M, Hermon C. Spontaneous Abortion
        And Work With Visual Display Units. British Journal Of Industrial
        Medicine 1992; 49:507–12

Ro93   Rouayrol JC, Rapport Sur Les Champs Electromagneticque De Tres
        Basse Frequence et. al.,. Sante (Report On Extremely Low-Frequen-
        cy Electromnagnetic Fields And Health). Bulletin De L'academie
        Nationale De Medicine 1993;177:1031–40

Ro94   Rosenbaum PF, Vena JE, Zielezny MA, And Michalek AM. Occupa-
        tional Exposures Associated With Male Breast Cancer. American
        Journal Of Epidemiology 1994;139:30-36

Sa86   Sander R, And Brinkmann J. Biological Effects Of Low Frequency
        Magnetic Fields. In: Berhnhardt JHG (Ed.) Biological Effects Of Stat-
        ic And Extremely Low Frequency Magnetic Fields. Proceedings Of
        The Symposium; 1985 May Neurenberg BGA Schriften 3/86. Mu-
        nich: MMV Medizin Verlag; 1986:113

Sa87   Savitz DA, And Calle EE. Leukemia And Occupational Exposure To
        Electromagnetic Fields: Review Of Epidemiologic Surveys, Journal
        Of Occupational Medicine. 1987;29:47–51

Sa88   Savitz D., Case-Control Study Of Childhood Cancer And Residen-
        tial Exposure To Electric And Magnetic Fields. Am J Epidemiol.
        1988;128:21–38

Sa89   Savitz DA, and Feingold L. Association of Childhood Cancer With
        Residential Traffic Density. Scandinavian Journal of Work and Envi-
        ronmental Health. 1989;15:360–363

Sa90a   Salzinger K, Freimark S, Mccullough M, et. al.,. Altered Operant Be-
        havior Of Adult Rats After Perinatal Exposure To 60 Hz Electromag-
        netic Fields. Bioelectromagnetics 1990;11:105–116

Sa90b   Savitz DA, And Chen J. Parental Occupation And Childhood Can-
        cer: Review Of Epidemiologic Evidence. Environmental Health
        Perspectives 1990;88:325–337

Sa90c   Savitz DA, John EM, And Kleckner RC. Magnetic Field Exposure
        From Electric Appliances And Childhood Cancer. 1990;131:763–773

Sa93a   Saffer JD, And Thurston SJ. Alteration Of Gene Expression By ELF
        Fields. (Abstract) Contractor's Review, Savannah, Georgia Novem-
        ber, 1993

Sa93b   Sahl JD, Kelsh MA, Greenland S. Cohort And Nested Case-Control
        Studies Of Hematopoietic Cancers And Brain Cancer Among Elec-
        tric Utility Workers. Epidemiology 1993;4:104–113

Sa93c   Savitz DA, Health Effects Of Low-Frequency Electric And Magnetic
        Fields. Environmental Science And Technology 1993;27:51–4

Sa94   Sarasua S, And Savitz D. Cured And Broiled Meat Consumption In
        Relation To Childhood Cancer:Denver, Colorado (UnitedStates)
        Cancer Causes and Control 1994;5:141–148

Sa95   Savitz DA, and Loomis DP. Magnetic Field Exposure in Relation to Leukemia and Brain Cancer Mortality Among Electric Utiility Workers. American Journal of Epidemiology. 1995;141:123–134

Sc82   Schottenfeld D, Fraumeni JF Jr. Cancer Epidemiology And Prevention. Philadelphia: W Saunders, 1982

Sc93   Schreiber GH, Swaen GMH, Meijers JMM, et.al. Cancer Mortality And Residence Near Electricity Transmission Equipment: A Retrospective Study. Int Journal Of Epidemiology 1993;22:9–15

Se88   Severson RK, Stevens RG, Kaune WT, Thomas DB, Heuser L, Davis S Sever LE. Acute Nonlymphocytic Leukemia And Residential Exposure To Power Frequency Magnetic Fields. Am J Epidemiol 1988;128:10–38

Sh93a   Shaw GM, And Croen L. Human Adverse Reproductive Outcomes And Electromagnetic Field Exposures: Review Of Epidemiologic Studies. Environmental Health Perspectives 1993;101:107–121

Sh93b   Shubik P, Pesticides And The Delaney Amendment (Letter To The Editor) Science 1993;260:1409

Si87   Sikov DN, Rommeriem JL, Beamer RL et. al.,. Developmental Studies Of Hanford Miniature Swine Exposed To 60-Hz Electric Fields. Bioelelectromagnetics 1987:8;229–42

Si93   Sitthi-Amorn C, And Poshyachinda V. Bias. The Lancet 1993;342:286–288

Sl90   Slovic P, Kraus N, And Covello VT What Should We Know About Making Risk Comparisons? Risk Analsysis 1990;10:389–92

Sm92   Smith GD, Phillips AN And Neaton JD Smoking As "Independent" Risk Factor For Suicide. Illustration Of An Artifact From Observational Epidemiology. Lancet 1992;340:709–712

Sm94   Smith RF, Clarke RL, And Justesen DR. Behavioral Study Of Rats To ELF Magnetic Fields. Bioelectromagnetics 1994;15:411–426

Sn49   Snow J, On Cholera, Harvard University Press, Cambridge, MA, 1949

So89   Sondik EJ. Progress In Cancer Prevention And Control, In Maulitz RC, (Ed.) Unnatural Causes: Three Leading Killer Diseases In America. New Brunswick, Rutgers University Press, 1989, pp. 111–134

Sp85   Spitz, M., Johnson, C. Neuroblastoma And Paternal Occupation: A Case-Control Analysis. Am J. Epidemiol 1985; 121:924–9

St88   Statistical Bulletin. Major Causes Of Accident Mortality Among Children: United States, 1988. Metropolitan Life Insurance Company. 1992;73:2–8

St87   Stevens RG, Electric Power And Breast Cancer: A Hypothesis. American Journal Of Epidemiology 1987;125:556–561

St89   Stuchly MA, And Lecuyer DW. Exposure To Electromagnetic Fields In Arc Welding. Health Physics 1989;56:297

St92a   Stevens RG, Davis S, Thomas DB et. al.,. Electric Power, Pineal Func-
         tion, And The Risk Of Breast Cancer. The FASEB Journal
         1992;6:853–860

St92b   Stuchly MA, Mclean JRN, Burnett M, et. al.,. Modification Of Tumor
         Promotion In The Mouse Skin By Exposure To An Alternating Field.
         Cancer Letters 1992; 65:1–7

Te89   Tenforde TS, Electroreception And Magneticoreception In Simple
         And Complex Organisms. Bioelectromagnetics 1989;10:215–221

Th86   Thomas Tl, Fontham ET, Norman SA, Stemhagen A, And Hoover
         RN. Occupational Risk Factors For Brain Tumors. Scand Journal
         Work Environmental Health 1986;12:121–127

Th88   Thompson RAE, Michaelson SM, And Nguyen QA. Influence Of
         60-Hz Magnetic Fields On Leukemia. Biolelectromagnetics
         1988;9:149–158

Th91   Theriault G. Health Effects Of Electromagnetic Fields On Workers:
         Epidemiologic Studies. In: Proceedings Of The Scientific Workshop
         On The Health Effects Of Electric And Magnetic Fields. January
         30–31, 1991 U.S. Department Of Health And Human Services, Pub-
         lic Health Service, Center For Disease Control, National Institute
         For Occupational Safety And Health, Dhhs (Niosh) Publication No.
         91–111 (Undated Publication)

Th93   Thomas DB. Breast Cancer In Men. Epidemiologic Reviews 1993;
         15:220–231

Th94   Theriault G, Goldberg M, Miller AB, et. al.,. Cancer Risks Associated
         With Occupational Exposure To Magnetic Fields Among Electric
         Utility Workers In Ontario And Quebec, Canada, And France:
         1970–1989. American Journal Of Epidemiology 1994;139:550– 572

To86   Tomenius, L., 50-Hz Electromagnetic Field Environment And The
         Incidence Of Childhood Tumors In Stockholm County. Bioelectro-
         magnetics. 1986;7(2):191–207

To90   Tomatis A (Ed) . Cancer: Causes, Occurrences, and Control. 1990 In-
         ternational Agency For Research on Cancer. Scientific Publications
         # 100. Oxford University Press, New York

Tr94   Trichopoulos D. Are Electric or Magnetic Fields Affecting Mortality
         From Breast Cancer in Women? Journal of the National Cancer Insti-
         tute. 1994;86:885–886

Ty90   Tynes T, And Anderson A. Electromagnetic Fields And Male Breast
         Cancer. (Letter) Lancet 1990;396:1596

Ty92   Tynes T, Andersen A. And Langmark F. Incidence Of Cancer In Nor-
         wegian Workers Potentially Exposed To Electromagnetic Fields.
         American Journal Of Epidemiology 1992;136:81–88

USC92   Electric And Magnetic Field Exposure, Chemical Exposure, And
         Leukemia Risk In "Electrical" Occupations. Prepared By The Uni-
         versity Of Southern California. EPRI Tr–101723, December 1992

VDT

Erickson A. (1986) An Epidemiological Study Of Work With Video Screens And Pregnancy Outcome: II. A Case-Control Study American Journal Of Industrial Medicine 9:459–75

Erickson A. (1986) An Epidemiological Study Of Work With Video Screens And Pregnancy Outcome I. A Registry Study. American Journal Of Industrial Medicine 9:447–57

Goldhaber MK, Polan MR and Hiatt RA. The risk of Miscarriage and Birth Defects among Women who Use Video Display Terminals Duuring Pregnancy. American Journal of Industrial Medicine 1988;13:695–706

Kurppa K. Birth Defects And Exposure To Video Display Terminals During Pregnancy. Scan Journal Work Environ Health 1985, 11:353–6

Mcdonald AD,(1988) Work With Visual Display Units In Pregnancy, British Journal Of Industrial Medicine 1988;45:509– 15

Nurminene T, And Kurppa K, Office Employment, Work With Video Display Terminals And Course Of Pregnancy. Scand Journal Work And Environmental Health 1988;14:293

Roman E, Beral V, Pelerin M, And Hermon C. Spontaneous Abortion And Work With Visual Display Units. British Journal Of Industrial Medicine 1992;49:507–512

Ve90   Vena JE, et. al.,. Use Of Electric Blankets And Risk Of Testicular Cancer. American Journal Of Epidemiology. 1990;131:759–762.

Ve91   Vena JE, Graham S, Hellmann R, et. al.,. Use Of Electric Blankets And Risk Of Postmenopausal Breast Cancer. American Journal Of Epidemiology 1991; 131:759–62

Ve93   Verkasalo PK, Pukkala E, Hongisto MY, Vlajus JE, Jarvinen PJ, Heikkila KY, And Koskenvuo M. Risk Of Cancer In Finnish Children Living Close To Power Lines. British Medical Journal 1993;307:895– 899

Wa92a   Walleczek J. Electromagnetic Field Effects On The Cells Of The Immune System: The Role Of Calcium Signalling. FASEB J. 1992;6:3177–3185

Wa92b   Waller R. quoted in article, Back To The Days Of Deadly Smogs. The New Scientist December 5, 1992, P25.

We79   Wertheimer N, And Leeper E. Electrical Wiring Configurations And Childhood Cancer. Am J Epidemiol 1979; 109:273–284

We80   Wertheimer N, Electrical Wiring Configurations And Childhood Leukemia In Rhode Island. Am J Epidemiol. 1980:111(4):461–2

We82   Wertheimer N, And Leeper E. Adult Cancer Related To Electrical Wires Near The Home. International Journal Of Epidemiology 1982;11:345–55

We86   Wertheimer N, Possible Effects Of Electric Blankets And Heated Waterbeds On Fetal Development. Biolectromagnetics 1986;7:13–22

We87   Wertheimer N, And Leeper N. Magnetic Field Exposure Related To Cancer Subtypes. Annals Of The New York Academy Of Sciences 1987;502:43–54

We89a   Wertheimer N., And Leeper E. Fetal Loss Associated With Two Seasonal Sources Of Electromagnetic Field Exposure. Brief Reports. Am J Epidemiol 1989; 129;220–224

We89b   Weinberg RA, Oncogenes And Tumor Suppressor Genes. In, Maulitz RC, (Ed.) Unnatural Causes, New Bruswick, Rutgers University Press, 1989 Pp. 83–93

We90   Weiss DS, Kirsneer R, And Eaglstein Wh. Electrical Stimulation And Wound Healing. Archives Of Dermatology 1990;126:222–225

We92   Wever RA, Circadian Rhythmicity Of Man Under The Influence Of Weak Electromagnetic Fields. In, Moore-Ede Mc, Campbell S, And Reiter RJ (Eds.) Electromagnetic Fields And Circadian Rhythmicity Birkhauser, Boston, 1992, pp 121–140

Wh86   Whitson GL, Carrier WL, Francis AA, et. al.,. Effects Of Extremely Low Frequency (ELF) Electric Fields On Cell Growth And DNA Repair In Human Skin Fibroblasts. Cell Tissue Kinetics 1986; 19:39–47

Wh93a   White D, Barge JM, George EA, And Riley K. The EMF Controversy And Reducing Exposure From Magnetic Fields. Interference Control Technologies, Inc. Gainesville, Va 1993

Wh93b   White P, Poison In Paradise, San Francisco Examiner. March 14, 1993

Wi88   Wilkins JR, Koutras RA. Paternal Occupation and Brain Cancer in Offspring: A Mortality Based Case Control Study. American Journal of Industrial Medicine, 1988;14:299–318

Wi90a   Wilson B, and Anderson LE, ELF Electromagnetic Field Effects on the Pineal Gland. In, Wilson, B., Stevens, R., And Anderson, L. (Eds.) Extremely Low Frequency Electromagnetic Fields: The Question Of Cancer. Batelle, Richland, 1990 pp157–186

Wi 90b Windham GC, Fenswter L, Swan SH, And Neutra RR. Use Of Video Display Terminals During Pregnancy And The Risk Of Spontaneous Abortion, Low Birthwigth, Or Intrauterine Growth Retardation. American Journal Of Industrial Medicine 1990;18:675–688

Wo93   Workshop On Statistics And Computing In Disease Clustering. Port Jefferson, New York, July 23–24, 1992. Proceedings Published In, Statistics In Medicine 1993;Number 19/20

Yo91   Youngson JHAM, Clayden AD, Myers A, And Cartright RAA. A Case- Control Study Of Adult Haematological Malignancies In Relation To Overhead Powerlines. British Journal Of Cancer 1991;63:977

Za93   Zaffanella L, Survey Of Residential Magnetic Field Sources. Final Report, Electric Power Research Institute, Palo Alto, California, 1993

Index